GREAT BODY THE FUN WAY

A complete body sculpting, fitness, and nutritional guide

INTEGRITY: the quality of being honest and
having strong moral principles; moral uprightness
"He is known to be a man of integrity"

Chris R. Rea

ReaShape

ISBN: 978-0-615-39392-6
reashape.com

The nutritional and health information in this book is based on the author's experiences. It is intended only as a guide and it not meant to replace the advice of a physician, dietician, physical therapist or other health professional. Always seek competent professional help if you have concerns about the appropriateness of this information for you.

Printed in the United States of America.

Contents

Acknowledgments

It's been a long career path, starting at age 14 with my high school wrestling coach, and now with the trainers, coaches and nutritionists who are currently providing me with their expertise. Thank you all. I would not be able to succeed without you.

– Chris Rea

Introduction

For all of you who have purchased this book from me, I personally want to say thank you. It truly excites me to help people achieve their fitness goals. For me, the ultimate reward I receive from working with people is results. It's all about the results, just as with everything else in life.

Results in fitness, believe it or not, is not the ultimate goal, rather it is only part of the ultimate goal. The other part is your daily well-being, because fitness will improve your quality of life in general. Many people overlook this and strictly wait for the results, looking just for a better physique. Only waiting for the results is the more difficult way to go about reaching your fitness goals. This long process can become very frustrating. This is where my system for getting into shape comes into play. In this book and others I will write, I will teach you my methods of getting into shape. Having fun and enjoying the moment is what it is all about.

I have helped many people achieve the body and health they wanted. My system changes for each individual person. Everyone is different and has different tastes in food and in training. People also have different goals they want to achieve with their bodies. This is why I treat each person on an individual basis, providing different workouts and meal plans for everyone. No two people are alike! Another way that I am different in my approach is that I place an emphasis on having fun by enjoying the workouts and meal plans as much as possible.

Getting into shape is like running a marathon. You want a constant steady pace that you can sustain throughout the entire journey.

Creating an enjoyable fitness regimen has an overall higher success rate. It's so much easier when you WANT to go to the gym and you WANT to eat that healthy meal instead of HAVING to go to the gym or HAVING to eat the healthy meal. Believe it or not, there is a much easier way to get into shape, and that's by having the most fun possible when you are eating right and exercising. Remember, we only live once, so why not live it to the max! All of your goals are within your grasp!

Do you all know the saying "Youth is wasted on the young?" My father used to tell me this all the time. What this saying really means is that it is such a waste to not reach your true potential and that time is in the essence. So follow your dreams, because they are attainable. Remember that dreams don't have expiration dates. Everyone has dreams, but only a few stay awake working to achieve them! Your time is now, because as of today you have 100 percent of your life left!

A Little About Myself

Hello everyone, my name is Christopher Rea. Most people call me Chris. Either one is fine for me. My family consisted of my father, Pepe Rea, my mother, Carmen Ramos Rea, and my brother Joe. My father immigrated to this country from Spain. My mother was born here, but her parents were both immigrants from Spain also. Believe it or not, our cultural backgrounds play a huge part in our lives. Growing up in the very diverse New York City region, I was always exposed to many different cultures in addition to the traditional Spanish culture in my home.

As a young boy I was very active, keeping myself busy in sports. By the time I was twelve years old I also had a job delivering newspapers. I was delivering at times two different newspapers, one in the early morning before school and the other at 3 p.m. right after school. The money I would save from working gave me money for game arcades and gasoline for my moped and spending money for the summer in Spain, where my parents would send me to live with my grandparents, uncle and aunt.

Summers in Spain were a big part of my life. I am so grateful that my parents, grandparents, uncles and aunts made the sacrifices they did for me. Going to Spain for the summer taught me things that would help me in fitness later on in life. The Mediterranean way of life, with its richness in food and quality of living, is something to admire. Siestas, seafood and wine should already tell you that Spain is a great place to live. There I would go spear gun fishing and live on the beach at my Tio Claudio and Tia Rosalina's house. On Samiera beach I had the best summers ever! Daily we kayaked and once a year we had our annual summer "Olympics." We all prepared by using corn stalks as hurdles and spears, big rocks as shot puts and BB guns for marksmanship. Swimming, running, everything! We had a blast. As a paper boy I was able to save enough money to buy a small boat and my father had bought me a small outboard motor. At thirteen years old I was going to different beaches in Spain, visiting friends and fishing. Every night after 11 p.m. because that's when the sun came down we would have a small bonfire at the beach and all of us would talk for a few hours. This was like a private beach with all the houses right on the sand. It was paradise. There were around twenty of us kids and we all had the greatest summers of our life! I still remain close to both Spain and the friendships I have there. During my grammar school years I played in all types of sports leagues, including baseball, basketball, football and soccer. Then came high school, where I became an Eagle Scout. I played soccer, track, tennis and wrestling. Playing sports and maintaining a part-time job at a Spanish restaurant kept my schedule filled. I was also involved with the school band, playing piano and saxophone, and many other school clubs and activities were part of my schedule. I entered high school at five feet tall and weighing only 100 pound. My freshman year, I wrestled in the 101-pound weight division. Being such a small kid would get me picked on once in a while but for some reason I knew that I would soon grow much bigger and that would prevent me from being picked on. As a freshman, I would tell the wrestling coach that I would probably be six feet tall and wrestle in the 188-pound division as a senior. Coach Kull laughed at me and said that five foot seven inches and 135 pounds was more realistic. He proved to be half right, because as a senior wrestling for my new coach, Dennis Hard, I wrestled at 135 pounds at five foot ten.

My first wrestling match was disastrous. I was pinned in less than two minutes! After the defeat I knew I had to make changes!

For Christmas that year, my mother bought me a weight set. At fourteen, I began lifting weights. The progress came slowly. The next year, I wrestled 115 pounds and at 122 pounds as a junior. When I was a high school junior is when people started noticing results with my body. The girls too began giving me a compliment or two and by my senior year I was sporting a six pack and won several wrestling championships. When wrestling ended, weight training would become a priority. By the time I graduated high school I weighed 175 pounds and everyone was noticing the changes! That's 40 pounds after wrestling season! My goal of six feet and 188 pounds now was becoming a reality.

I went on to wrestle in college in the 177-pound division as a freshman, then as a sophomore, junior and senior I grew to six feet and wrestled in the 190-pound division and finally reached my goal. Now I began feeling like me. The gains I made on my body were attributed to hard work, training and eating well. My college wrestling career would be interrupted from time to time because I had transferred schools several times. Finally, I ended up wrestling for a few different universities and becoming a two-time NCAA All-American wrestler in the 190-pound division. An All-American means that you placed in the top eight of all the universities and colleges in the entire country. Placing fourth and seventh in the U.S.A. was largely thanks to weight training and nutrition. My last year of college wrestling I was twenty nine year old and still I kept improving on my wrestling and body. As the oldest guy and an All-American on the team, I felt no different from everyone else during the practices and competition thanks to my weight lifting and meal regimen.

During my lengthy college career I also competed in several bodybuilding competitions either wiing or placing high in several of them. Being a competitive bodybuilder taught me a lot more about being shape, how to get in shape and how to maintain it. After college, I competed in the New York Golden Gloves boxing tournament as well as other boxing, wrestling, jiu jitsu and mixed martial arts (MMA) fights. Whether as an eighteen-year-old college fresh-man, a 29-year-old college senior, or as an older and more experienced athlete, I prepared for matches the same way. As a 34- and 35-year-old competitor in the New York Golden Gloves, I fought in the 201-pound division. Then I extended my career longer by competing and winning in MMA fights into my forties. Winning my last MMA fight felt no different than being 25, because I pretty much used the same training regimen.

Today, I maintain the same regimen, but every so often I make slight adjustments because I learn new techniques through both education and trial and error. Having an understanding of European culture, food and lifestyle and with an athletic background, I have combined the best of these experiences. I have managed to exercise and eat right everywhere imaginable, ranging from the rain forest in Brazil to gyms all over the world and even public parks in Mexico and Spain. Let's just say that I've come a long way from the 101-pound freshman in high school. So much has happened since and so much more will happen in the future. I have always been an action type of guy, always on the move, always looking for the next adventure. You can say that I am an adrenaline junky, but most of my sanity and stability I owe to both my upbringing and to exercise. All of us have that little spark in us to take on challenges and wanting to fulfill lifelong dreams. What a better way to start by getting into shape? Training and dieting will make you feel that little extra out of life, the feeling of thriving instead of just surviving.

So this is the concept I really want to teach people: Have fun WHILE getting into shape or MAINTAINING your shape so you can THRIVE!

Still, I have so much more to learn. Each day as I learn I enjoy sharing my knowledge and helping people. I really love this—it's my passion and my life!

Chapter 1: A New Beginning

Why do we want a healthier life? There are so many reasons we want to feel and look healthier, but we all need some type of push. Some of us need more than others! Trust me when I say this, because we all do!

I have been in training as a competitive athlete most of my life and not a day passes by when I don't feel like exercising and or eating properly. Throughout my career, I have realized that the results won't come overnight. However, what I have recently learned is that satisfaction will occur daily, especially after each workout. Enjoy the journey of achieving your fitness goals, because the process of healthy living is extremely rewarding and pleasant. Being in shape makes you feel healthy and pleased with your body. Health is something that everybody wants but money cannot buy this. It's achieved only through dedication and discipline.

Remember that there is no substitute for hard work. I have had so much more fulfillment in life thanks to being healthy. These small daily sacrifices and variations render huge benefits with zero drawbacks! If at any time during the course of this book, there is something you don't understand or have any questions, please contact me. I would be honored to help see to it that you reach your goals, 24/7. I will answer you back personally if you contact me at

If you want to look better, feel better, decrease stress, increase energy and have a happier mood, then let's begin! Just show me the will and I will show you the way! Because that's all it is—you must have the will to succeed, to endure, to persevere, to not be denied from reaching your fitness goals and the look you want! Remember that being shape and having great health is something that everyone wants! And I mean EVERYONE! A lot of people, but not everyone, want that gorgeous mansion or that beautiful Ferrari sports car, but some people would rather live in a low-key way, under the radar. However, not a single person out there will ever say they don't want to be in better shape, or they don't want to lose their fat legs, or put a little bit of muscle on their skinny arms, or have better endurance. Rich or poor, old or young, EVERYBODY wants a great body!

There's good news! A better body is very possible! And easier and faster than you can imagine! I may not know a lot of things, but I do know fitness, 100 percent! I'll give it to you straight, to the point, effectively and precisely.

Follow my ways and you will create a better and healthier body, I will promise you this. I am extremely confident in my work. But most of all, we will enjoy the process of getting in shape! I will make it so much more fun!

Let's get started!

Chapter 2: Tools of the Trade

As an Eagle Scout, our motto was "be prepared." This applies to every single area of life. Can a fisherman go fishing without his bait? Of course not! You can't get into great shape unprepared either. Cooking, training and rest are the three pieces of the puzzle of creating a great body. Buying the proper kitchen appliances will make your meal preparing a breeze. Buying a comfortable bed will ease your rest and a gym membership will facilitate your body-sculpting process. Please, by no means feel overwhelmed by thinking this is such a tremendous commitment. See it instead as a stepping-stone that will facilitate the process of getting into the best shape of your life!

Ever since I was a high school athlete on the wrestling team I have been studying nutrition and training. I'm always finding new and better ways to help the body reach its peak performance through nutritional and training techniques. Some of us may have the convenience of eating at home, while others may often have to eat away from home. Eating right in both situations will lead you toward the progress that you are looking to achieve.

In this chapter we are building a solid foundation right from the beginning so you will have the proper start toward your journey to getting into shape. With a solid foundation, you add security to the progress you're making, which then dramatically increases the success rate. Trust me when I say this. Over all the years that I have consistently stayed in shape, I have learned easier techniques every year. I'm now to the point where the process of getting into shape just continues to get easier as well as be more fun. Years ago, I absolutely hated the process of getting into shape. That led me to be not as happy throughout the day, which would always lead to either quitting the entire process or getting into great shape but not keeping it for long. That approach was just too grueling for me. In order to succeed in anything , you must enjoy what you do.

It's completely understandable that dieting and training may not be the most enjoyable activity for most people. That's why I developed a meal plan and exercise routine that will be the best, most enjoyable and easiest to follow for not only the short-term but the long-term as well. Having fun while training I believe is a fantastic approach. It has worked wonders for the clients I have trained and guided into getting into shape. It really is a wonderful system.

Proper kitchen appliances facilitate the process of getting you into shape. With the proper equipment becoming fit is that much easier. Think of a mechanic. How much more difficult would it be for him to repair cars if he didn't have the proper tools? Eagle Scouts, like me, follow the same motto, be prepared.

Home Chef

Being a home chef means that you are in a great position, because you know exactly what is in your food. Cooking at home will tremendously benefit your physique because it is the best option for eating the right foods for your health and your physique. When you cook at home, you can cook with the best ingredients possible while using the appliances of your choice. Personally, I truly enjoy having easy-to-use kitchen appliances. Keep it simple is another of my mottos. When you have the luxury of preparing your meals in the comfort and convenience of your own home, the sky is the limit for your nutrition. You can really dial in right down to the wire exactly which foods are going into your body—the quality, quantity and freshness. You will be surprised how easy and fun it is to prepare your own food. Another perk is if you cook for your date, he or she will truly be amazed by how you are not only self-sufficient but also health conscious about your body. Basically, they are looking at you as a pool of great genetics for having their children! Then again, let's not get ahead of ourselves but every man or woman wants the healthiest, strongest genes for their baby!

Appliances and Other Basic Items to Purchase

- Set of measuring cups and spoons (under $5)
- 9-inch frying pan
- Indoor electric cooking grill (around $50)
- Food scale, either digital or analog (around $20)
- Food steamer, either a steaming tray that fits inside a pot or separate electric steamer (from $7 to $35)
- Blender (around $20 to $100)
- Quart-size Ziploc bags (around $4 for 50 bags)
- Plastic containers in various sizes (around $2 to $20)
- Can opener (around $15 for an electric one)
- Utensils such as knives, cooking spoons, spatula, strainer, ladle (a few dollars or less apiece)
- Plastic cutting board (around $7)
- Microwave oven (around $35 to $100)

These home chef tools and appliances will definitely make your cooking experience a lot easier. They're not expensive and they last a long time. Also, you'd be surprised at the high-quality cooking utensils and appliances you can find inexpensively at a yard sale or church bazaar.

It's always a good practice to prepare several meals at once and store the other meals to eat later on. Preparing one or three meals takes the same time, so why not cook several at once? I cook just about every day, but I always cook three meals at once. For example, I might sauté three portions of chicken breast in the same frying pan and cook three sweet potatoes in the microwave. After eating one meal, I then save the other two meals in two separate quart-sized reclosable bags so I can take them with me when I am out for the rest of the day. Efficiency and simplicity is the key! When you go that extra mile to prepare your meals and carry them with you, it will definitely show in your physique and energy level. Your physique will look leaner and tighter because you have less bloat from water retention. Proper nutrition is the one of the secrets behind creating the fit body of your dreams. Without the right foods your body will not respond in the way you would want it to. When you cook for yourself, you have complete control over what you eat.

The Traveler

The traveler is always out and on the road, so of course eating out is part of the program. By buying and keeping a few items with you or in your car, eating right will be a lot easier for you. You won't be eating fast food or junk food instead of good food you made yourself. At first, eating properly at all times may seem like a drag, but it's one of the best investments that you can make.

Packing lightweight, already prepared food has always been a great way for me to eat right while traveling. My favorites are the three- to six-ounce pouches of tuna, salmon and chicken breast that you can get at the supermarket. These are great emergency meals that can be stored in your car trunk, your handbag, briefcase, or luggage. They don't need to be refrigerated and they're very convenient. Nothing feels better than eating a healthy meal like that when you are on a train, bus, airplane or even driving a car. Whey protein isolate powder is a fantastic choice while traveling. It is compact enough to bring with you everywhere and with just a little bit of water you can quickly make a tasty shake.

These emergency meals will come in handy from time to time. Emergency meals are to be eaten when it happens to be mealtime for you but you're be stuck in traffic, on a delayed flight, or when there are no healthy meal options available. Remember what the great football coach Vince Lombardy said, "Fatigue makes cowards of us all." What he meant was that when an athlete starts getting tired he/she begins to fall apart and lose. Now let's replace hungry with fatigue. When you're training and dieting and you become excessively hungry, you mentally break down and start to binge eat. That's terrible for your body and sabotages the dieting you're doing to achieve a lean body. Oftentimes you can't help binge eating, because your body is craving calories to be stored as fat to be used at a later time. Eating the right foods all day long and at the right times will keep you from becoming very hungry or having low blood sugar (hypoglycemia), which is what gives you the sugar and carbohydrate cravings.

You never want your body to get to this point. To prevent this you need to provide your body with a small and steady stream of high-quality nutrients. You must eat nutritious foods every two to four hours. I don't mean a four-course meal every two hours. Instead, eat moderate amounts of healthy foods, consuming just enough to satisfy your hunger and keep up your energy level. You will discover the right amounts for you with a little experimentation.

In addition to having a good food supply always handy while traveling, I recommend being prepared in other ways. Pack workout clothing so that regardless of where you are, you will be prepared to work out. If you always travel by car, make sure you put a gym bag in your trunk packed with a pair of sneakers, shorts/sweats and a t-shirt/sweatshirt. Traveling light has always been my motto. Take the bare minimum with you, because the extra gear isn't really needed.

Having a membership in a gym with a lot of locations is recommended but not necessary. I have devised many exercise routines that can be performed without having to be at a gym. Training in a gym is always preferred, of course, because you can always find the right equipment there. Also, being in an atmosphere where other people are training is definitely a motivator.

Chapter 3: Introduction to Healthy Foods and Meals

Cooking at home is perfect because you have so many different meal options to choose from. Stocking your food pantry with only quality food is a great way to insure that only the healthiest ingredients will go into your food.

Shopping for the right foods is where it all begins. Having only healthy food in your house will really set the pace and give you a solid foundation toward getting that nice physique. To use myself as an example, in my house there is only healthy food available for me to eat. Keeping a healthy food supply prevents me from binge eating and cheating on my diet by eating the wrong foods, such as cookies, cakes, bacon, and so on. If these foods aren't in the house, but good, healthy choices are, it's a lot easier to eat right.

Hey, I am only human, I have weaknesses too. Every so often I break down and cheat a little on my diet, so the healthier the food is in my house, the less damage to my physique will occur during a binge, a cheat, or a breakdown in my diet. This is called damage control. Think of a recovering alcoholic or drug addict. It's not safe for them to be around bars or anywhere else drugs and alcohol are readily available. Even the people you associate with make a big difference. If your friends are in shape, you are more likely to follow your regimen to keep up with them. But if you are constantly around out-of-shape people , you may become complacent and give in by slacking off on your meal and training regimen. A lot of psychology is behind this. It's all mental.

A simple trip to the supermarket can be your true savior, because pretty much anything and everything healthy is available there. Buying fresh "real" food, meaning food that is not already Prepared, is the best way to go. Fresh turkey breast, fish, lean cuts of meat, fresh fruit and vegetables are foods that will really take your body and health to new levels. Once prepared properly, these ordinary supermarket foods will be the secret to looking and feeling fantastic. Even for those of you who think you're not a good chef, you're in for a big surprise. It's so much easier than you think to prepare nutritious and delicious meals. Don't worry at all, because later on in this book there is an entire section that is dedicated to easy recipes for the home chef. Right now, I'm writing just a little about food and cooking because a little knowledge now will get you ready for much more knowledge about cooking in the upcoming chapters.

So now let's start with a simple list of which foods to buy, how to prepare them, and when eat.

Supermarket Food Shopping List
- Chicken breast
- Turkey breast
- Wild-caught fish
- Fish in a can or pouch
- Liquid egg whites
- Whey protein isolate
- Soy protein isolate
- Omega 3 eggs
- Fresh fruit
- Vegetables (fresh, frozen or canned)
- Unsalted almonds
- Unsalted walnuts
- Extra virgin olive oil
- Canola oil or olive oil cooking spray
- Avocados

- Sweet potatoes
- Brown rice
- Whole-grain pasta
- Whole-grain high-fiber bread
- Whole-grain high-fiber wraps
- Old-fashioned oats
- Oat bran
- Bran cereal
- Unprocessed wheat bran

These are the food basics. There are more foods that also qualify as optimum performance foods as well. Please let me know if there is a particular food you would like to know more about. I do know a decent amount about food shopping because I really love going supermarkets to walk through the aisles and read the labels on all of the food. (I love going to hardware stores too—I really like tools.) Being in a supermarket is an education and challenge for me. Each time I go shopping I read new food labels and always try to find a healthier version of the foods that I had purchased before. It's a great feeling when sometimes I find a new great food or brand that I never knew before. I love to try new foods that will facilitate my body-improving process.

If you're traveling for whatever reason—business or pleasure— that means you're not able to eat at home or work out at your regular fitness center. In this chapter I will only give you a brief and simple introduction on how to stay in great shape without the comfort of your own home or fitness center. Later on in this book, I will really get into the entire body-improving process for someone who is always out on the road or on vacation. For now, let's plant the seed in your head on how to have a great body without the comfort of home or your regular fitness center.

The Traveler

Being on the road is never easy. Traveling makes it even harder to keep up the healthiest lifestyle. There are a few staple foods that will really make your travel/driving experience as healthy as can be. Back to the old Scouts motto, "Be prepared." Wherever you go or may be, if you have the right foods with you, your body will not pay the price at all. In fact, you will still be able to maintain or even improve your body. For a person like myself, who is rarely at home, eating right and exercising is still always a part of my agenda.

Throughout the years I've been able to put together high-quality meals that are small, compact, inexpensive and highly nutritious. Granted, we all have different tastes in foods and preferences, such as being a vegetarian, so I have compiled an option for each of these categories.

Ideal "Carry Along" Foods

These are the foods that I most frequently bring with me wherever I go. They are convenient and can be eaten with little or no preparation.

- 2.5- to 7-ounce pouches of tuna, salmon and chicken breast
- Rice cakes (plain)
- Whey protein isolate
- Soy protein isolate
- Powdered egg whites
- Raw vegetables
- Raw fruits
- Unsalted almonds
- Unsalted walnuts
- Dehydrated fruits
- Dehydrated vegetables

Chapter 4: Introduction to Eating Efficiently

Now you're starting to see my whole fitness concept. I slowly but surely take you through the steps towards creating that nice body that you always wanted. Eating healthy is an extremely important step.

There are so many ways to eat healthy and prepare balanced meals. I will simply list a few examples here to help get you started. Meal combinations should be chosen to your taste. If you don't like some of the foods I suggest, substitute other healthy choices. Try to vary your meal choices and mix up the combinations so you don't get bored and tempted to go off the plan.

Remember, you will be doing a lot of eating. Pick the meals that will be easiest for you to continue eating properly, with as little junk food cravings as possible. In my years involved in fitness, I've seen a lot of different diets come and go. People start and stop new diets constantly, because the diets are hard to stick with. The knowledge that I have gathered from experience has proved to be quite effective in sticking to an effective meal plan as effortlessly as possible. It's much easier to stick with than a fad diet.

Foods are broken down into three basic groups: proteins, carbohydrates (either simple or complex) and fats. Proteins are foods such as meat, poultry, and fish. Simple carbohydrates are refined starchy foods such as white flour, white bread, and pasta. These foods are fast-acting—they enter your bloodstream quickly and raise your blood sugar. Complex carbohydrates are slow-acting foods such as sweet potatoes, whole-grain bread, and brown rice. These foods have more natural fiber in them and take longer to digest. They don't hit your body with a big spike of blood sugar. Fats fall into several categories. Monounsaturated and polyunsaturated fats, such as olive oil, canola oil, and the fat found naturally in nuts and avocados are the healthy fats. Trans fats (partially hydrogenated vegetable oil), which are found in many processed foods, and saturated fat, which are found in meat and dairy products, are the unhealthy fats.

When preparing meals, your fitness goals must be taken into consideration. Do you want to lose, maintain or gain weight? There are many healthy foods and meal combinations that will help you achieve your fitness goals. Choose the ones that taste and work best for you.

Food Categories

Protein
Chicken breast
Turkey breast
Fish (wild-caught or canned)
London broil
Egg whites
Whey protein isolate
Soy protein isolate

Carbohydrates (starches)
Brown rice
Whole-grain pasta
Old-fashioned oats
Oat bran
Bran cereal
Sweet potato
Wild rice

Fiber
Fruits
Vegetables

Fats
Almonds
Peanuts
Olive oil
Egg yolk
Coconut
Avocado
Canola oil
Olive oil

This is a basic food table that I follow to properly combine food in order to create well-balanced meals. To get you started on the right track, I made it pretty easy for everyone to understand.

In the later chapters, there will be more a more comprehensive format on nutrition. Easing you into it is my most effective approach. Keep telling yourself that getting into shape is more like a marathon than a 100 meter sprint. Like a marathon runner, you must maintain a comfortable pace so you can stick with it in the long run.

Now that we are learning about healthy food, we must take the next step and combine them in a way that best suits your fitness goals, lifestyle and taste. Food combinations will vary
depending on your goals—whether you want to lose, maintain or gain weight. Do you want to lose body fat/body weight only? Do you want to gain muscle mass while losing body fat? Maintain your current weight while losing body fat and gaining muscle? Depending on your goal, you will select different meal options. Fortunately, the combinations work for all types of people, even if they have entirely different goals on how they want their body to look, feel and perform. A few examples will show you what this all actually means.

Meal Option Examples
To Lose Body Fat/Body Weight:
For each meal, choose 1 protein with 1 fiber.

Examples of body fat/body weight reduction meals:
Breakfast
1 cup liquid egg whites (spray oil on frying pan)
1 banana

Dinner
6 ounces London broil
Steamed spinach (as much as you want)

To Lose Body Fat/Increase Muscle Mass:
For each meal, choose 1 protein, 1 carbohydrate, 1 fiber, 1 fat (fat is not required if eating meat or fish as protein)

Examples of body fat/increase muscle mass meals:
Breakfast
1 cup liquid egg whites, 1 whole egg (spray oil on frying pan)
½ cup old-fashioned oats cooked with water (add zero calorie sweetener if you wish)
½ cup blueberries

Dinner
6 ounces broiled fish
1 cup brown rice
1 green salad with oil and vinegar dressing

I have given you four examples of well-balanced meals. Now, let's look at two examples of two days of well-balanced meals, one day for each desired goal, whether it's body fat reduction or body fat reduction with increasing muscle mass. A complete day's worth of optimum nutrition is listed below. There are many more meal combinations that will work efficiently if the listed meals are not suited for you. This is a simple transition to get you headed on the right track.

Meal Day for Body Fat Reduction
Breakfast (7 A.M.)
1 cup egg whites (spray oil on frying pan)
1 cup strawberries

Snack (10 A.M.)
1 cup nonfat Greek yogurt

Lunch (1 P.M.)
1 can or pouch light tuna in water with small green salad (oil and vinegar dressing)

Mid-afternoon Snack (4 P.M.)
1 scoop whey protein isolate with water
1 apple

Dinner (7 P.M.)
5 ounces baked chicken breast
Steamed vegetables

Bedtime snack (only if you are hungry)
1 cup egg whites (spray oil on frying pan)

Drink 2 to 4 quarts water daily.

Coffee and tea in the morning if you wish.

Meal Day for Body Fat Reduction While Increasing Muscle Mass
Breakfast (7 A.M.)
1 cup egg whites plus 1 whole egg (spray oil on frying pan)
⅓ cup oat bran
1 banana

Snack (10 A.M.)
1 cup nonfat Greek yogurt

Lunch (1 P.M.)
5 ounces baked chicken breast on whole wheat bread with lettuce and tomato

Mid-afternoon Snack (4 P.M.)
1 scoop whey protein isolate
1 tablespoon all-natural peanut butter

Dinner (7 P.M.)
5 ounces broiled fish
1 cup whole-grain pasta
Green salad (oil and vinegar dressing)

Bedtime snack (only if you are hungry)
1 cup egg whites and 1 whole egg (spray oil on frying pan)

There are many more meal combinations that can be provided for you. The best meals are the ones that most complement your taste and lifestyle.

Another important factor is the amount of times per day to eat and at what time to eat. Eating every two to four hours is necessary in order to lose body fat and/or gain muscle mass. Frequent eating helps speed metabolism and provides efficient digestion. Eating balanced and frequent meals is extremely important for several reasons. Due to the smaller amount of food at each meal your stomach eventually shrinks in capacity to accommodate to the smaller meals. You become full with much less food. Think of the gas tank in a small car: it takes less fuel to fill but it empties much quicker, requiring more frequent refueling. Another added benefit to balanced and frequent meals is your blood sugar stays steady. Big meals with a lot of carbohydrates make your body produce spikes of insulin, the hormone that carries blood sugar into your cells. Smaller, regular meals with small amounts of carbohydrates keep your insulin steady, not overloaded. Insulin spikes cause sleepiness and an uncomfortable overeating feeling. That leads to being immobile for at least an hour after eating—and that means you're being unproductive, wasting time, etc. Nobody wants to feel overly full, bloated and lazy at any time. At first, when you begin to reduce your portion size you will constantly feel hungry. That's only because your "stretched out" stomach will feel empty with the smaller portions. This feeling of hunger is only temporary. With every healthy meal that you eat your stomach will keep reducing itself until it is so small that now with the smaller meal you feel satisfied.

At the beginning , do not hesitate to eat if you feel hungry, as you probably will. In fact, I urge you eat a healthy meal whenever you feel hungry. Don't worry about eating too many times a day. As long as the portions are small and the meals are healthy, your body will simply burn through them while making your metabolism speed up at the same time. Small and frequent meals will dramatically improve your body's ability to burn fat and at the same time build lean muscle mass. If you're a woman, don't be scared about building too much muscle mass—your hormones will keep you from getting too bulky. Instead, you'll look strong and toned (I'll explain about the hormones later on). For both women and men, building muscle not only strengthens your body but increases your metabolism as well, enabling your body to burn more fat and be more alert and energized throughout the day.

Eating smaller, more frequent meals during the day keeps you energized all day long with no post-meal downtime. That means being more active and having more energy to do the things you like without that uncomfortable "stuffed" feeling. Using myself as an example, I prepare three meals at once which takes approximately 15 minutes and eat throughout the day while walking, driving, riding a bicycle, etc. People often say that they don't have the time to cook their meals. I tell them to give me a minute so we can do the math. Cost, time, quality cooking wins in all three categories! Unanimous decision victory! Let me explain by category.

Cost
1 self-prepared 5-ounce chicken breast costs $1.80.
1 small sweet potato costs 60 cents.

This equals around $2.40 for a high-quality fresh meal. The same meal purchased at a deli or restaurant would be at least $6.

The winner is self-prepared meals!

Time
Preparing three meals takes 15 minutes, or 5 minutes per meal.

Buying a meal at a restaurant takes approximately 10 to 15 minutes for take-out and much longer for table service.

The winner is self-prepared meals!

Quality
When you cook for yourself you can choose the freshness and quality. Take-out or restaurant food is a gamble, because you can't really be sure of the quality and freshness. Also, restaurant portion sizes are large, meaning you can easily overeat without realizing it. Another factor is that we tend to eat more and more of the foods we are not supposed to eat when we don't prepare our own food.

The winner is self-prepared meals!

Regardless of how you look at it, all roads lead to self-prepared meals. Cook for yourself and without question it will show in your physique. You will achieve your goals faster and more economically!

Chapter 5: Introduction to Efficient Eating, At Home or Out

Perhaps I may seem redundant on the topic of nutrition, but proper eating is extremely important for looking, feeling and performing better. Achieving your physical goals relies on three variables that are equally important. Think of a tripod that holds a video camera. It has three legs and each leg is equally important for the camera to remain up. If one leg is removed, the camera falls! Achieving your physical goals is like a tripod: one leg is nutrition, another is exercise and the other leg is rest. Each are worth 33 percent of your fitness goals: exercise, nutrition, rest. Doubling up on training and foregoing the rest, or doubling up on nutrition while forgoing training, won't work. In fact, this is a recipe for failure! Let's not forget these three legs of the tripod and how all three work together! I will provide healthy examples of efficient eating for you, whether you are on the road, only have access to fast food, or can eat self-prepared meals

Fast Food Restaurants
McDonald's
Two McGrill sandwiches without the bread
Garden salad with no or low-calorie dressing
Water, diet soda, coffee, tea without milk and with zero calorie sweetener

Chinese
Steamed shrimp with vegetables (no MSG)

Water, diet soda
Diner
Broiled fish with steamed vegetables, garden salad, oil and vinegar dressing
Water, diet soda, coffee, tea without milk and with zero calorie sweetener

Japanese restaurant
Salad
Sashimi or steamed seafood with seaweed

Applebee's or other fast-casual restaurant
Grilled chicken breast, steamed vegetables, garden salad, oil and vinegar dressing
Water, diet soda, coffee, tea without milk and with zero calorie sweetener

High-End Restaurants
Shrimp cocktail or clams on the half shell for appetizer; Steamed lobster, steamed vegetables, garden salad, oil and vinegar dressing; fresh fruit for dessert

As you can see, these are just a few meal options for eating healthy while eating out. By giving you a few examples now and many more later in this book, I believe you'll easily come to understand this. Taking small baby steps is the right approach for success in getting into shape.

Cooking at Home
Preparing your own healthy meals to go is another fantastic approach toward reaching your fitness goals. Simple and quick carry meals can provide the right nutrition quickly and economically.

Cooking at home will become easier as you read along so don't worry one bit. By the time you finish reading this book, you will be a well-equipped chef!

Introduction to Home-Cooked Carry Meals

Meal #1
5 ounces baked chicken breast
1 cup brown rice
1 fruit

Bag the chicken and rice in a quart-sized Ziploc bag with a paper towel to absorb the moisture and oil.

Meal #2
1 can or pouch salmon
1 cucumber, sliced
Fruit

Bag the salmon and cucumber in a quart-sized Ziploc bag with a paper towel to absorb the moisture and oil.

Meal #3
Egg white omelet
Raw or cooked pepper strips
Fruit

Bag the omelet and pepper in a quart-sized Ziploc bag with a paper towel to absorb the moisture and oil.

What to Drink?
Keep at least a quart and preferably a gallon of water in your car at all times. This is a great habit, because it will enable you to sip water

all day long, to your body's benefit. Water is something that you can't have enough. It's free from your sink, it has zero calories, and it flushes out your body. Bloating from water retention can often be our worst nightmare. Surprisingly, drinking plenty of water will actually keep you from retaining water by flushing out your body's impurities. Your skin will look better too.

Chapter 6: Introduction to Simple Exercises

The number one question people ask me about exercising is, "Which exercises are the best?" My answer is always "The ones you like!"

In other words, every exercise is good. What makes an exercise great for you is that you enjoy it. If the time you spend exercising is pleasant, achieving your physical goals will be so much easier. Exercises vary from running, weight training, basketball, to calisthenics and many more options, such as playing tennis or riding a bike. By the way, fishing and darts don't count, so don't join any darts or fishing leagues instead of joining a gym!

Resistance exercise such as weight training and calisthenics differ from cardiovascular exercise such as running and basketball, which make your heart beat faster. Resistance training works by building muscle mass, which leads to increased overall metabolism. Resistance training burns fewer calories than cardiovascular exercise during each training session. However, you burn more calories overall throughout the day, because after resistance training your body is working to repair the muscle tissue. That's how muscles grow and become stronger—they tear during training, then repair themselves to become larger and stronger. The repair process takes approximately 48 hours per muscle, so that equals an additional 48 hours of increased metabolism! Your body metabolism increases whenever the body is working. An increased metabolism allows you to eat more food without gaining body fat! As an example, think of two cars that are same except under the hood. A Ford Mustang with a six-cylinder engine burns less gas than the same car with an eight-cylinder engine. On the outside, both cars are identical, but the eight cylinder uses more fuel and is more powerful than the six cylinder.

That's your body with and without muscles. With muscles, your body is more powerful and burns more calories throughout the day, requiring more food intake than your body without the muscles and weight training!

You can incorporate cardiovascular exercise into your resistance training routine by not resting between sets (I will explain about super-setting later on). Cardiovascular training by itself is great for your heart's strength and blood circulation. The truth is that all training is great! Now let me show you some quality workouts so we can begin!

Calisthenics: Working Out Without Weights

Let's begin by learning how to work out without weight equipment. Instead, you'll use your own body weight. Believe it or not, some of the best physiques I have seen were from plain old push-ups and pull-ups, which use just your natural body weight. If for a moment you are questioning the effectiveness of calisthenics, simply look at an Olympic gymnast's physique. See how muscular and lean they are? That's all from just moving their own body weight. Another advantage to performing calisthenics and body weight exercises is that your body will hold onto the muscles you develop. If, for some reason you had to stop training, your body will stay fit for a longer time.

Body Weight Calisthenics Workout

Monday and Thursday
5 sets wide grip pull-ups (each set is 9 to 12 reps)
5 sets push-ups (20 reps)
3 sets close grip chin-ups (9 to 12 reps)
3 sets dips (10 to 15 reps)
Super-set all 4 sets

Wednesday
1 hour cardio of your choice: bike ride, jog or run, brisk walk, play a sport

Tuesday and Friday
7 sets walking lunges (15 yards)
7 sets free squats (20 reps)
5 sets standing calf raises (20 reps)
Super-set all 3 sets
Saturday and Sunday

Partial time off: Engage in a leisurely activity such as walking, playing with kids and family, walking, sightseeing, bowling, fishing, playing Frisbee, softball, golf, handball, or any other activity you enjoy.

Resistance Training Weekly Workout (at a gym)

Monday and Thursday
5 sets inclined bench press (8 to 12 reps)
5 sets T-bar rows (6 to 8 reps)
3 sets dumbbell bench press (9 to12 reps)
3 sets lat pull-downs (10 to12 reps)
100 crunches

All sets are super-setted.

Wednesday
1 hour cardio of your choice: bike ride, jog or run, brisk walk, play a sport

Tuesday and Friday
3 sets leg extension (8 to12 reps)
3 sets leg curls

3 sets lunges (15 yards)
3 sets stiff-legged dead lifts
3 sets barbell squats
3 sets standing calf raises
50 sit-ups

All sets are super-setted.

These are just two simple examples of resistance training. One can be at a gym and the other could be anywhere—a park, gym, home, hotel, etc. I will teach you many more exercise techniques and diets later on in this book, because it is important to ease into everything that I am teaching you. These training methods are not short-term. Rather, they're a long-term lifestyle. The example I use is, this is not a 100 meter sprint , it's a marathon! We must work together to custom-build a training and diet regimen that is 100 percent tailor-made for you— your needs, goals, lifestyle, etc. This is a long-term commitment that in order for you to more easily achieve your fitness goals!

Just think of me as your virtual personal trainer and nutritionist. I will constantly adjust your regimen according to your progress, goals and lifestyle changes. Constantly modifying your training and diet along the way is very important for achieving success. You want to dialed in precisely and specifically for you! Enjoy the ride toward achieving the body you have long desired. I will see to it that every step of the way will be as pleasant and enjoyable as possible!

Remember that as the class clown, I am a strong believer in having fun. Sometimes I may have a little too much fun, but that's OK. I strongly believe that having fun is not only a great motivator but a great way to go about your daily life and, of course, your exercise routine. Believe it or not, there is a fun way to get into shape. Being in shape is definitely a lot of fun but getting into shape is always the part that everyone dislikes. Why not change the workout and diet often, until we find the best, most fun and easiest combination for you to follow? It is possible! I am living it and many of my clients are as well.

The basis of my methods is called "effective fun." Now you can mix business with pleasure, because you will be getting into shape and having fun at the same time. Who wouldn't want that! Don't get me wrong—it's not that easy, because work, discipline and dedication will be involved. Still, it will be much more pleasant because we add fun into the mix. Trust me, there is no better or effective way to getting into shape!

Chapter 7: Putting It All Together

For you to turn your fitness dreams into reality as simply as possible, I have created a formula that makes the body-transforming process so user-friendly that anyone can successfully do this. Why makes me so sure? Because I have vast experience in achieving fitness goals myself and guiding many others through the process of achieving their fitness goals as well. Of course, there are many informative diet/exercise books found on shelves of book stores and libraries. Are they any good? I am sure many of them are. There are many knowledgeable people writing fitness books today. I would like you to read as many of them as possible, because the more you read the more knowledge you will acquire. I've myself have learned a lot from reading nutrition and fitness books. You may like a certain author's methods more than mine. That's quite all right with me. We all need to feel that chemistry that a coach can provide for us, so I would be extremely happy for you if you were to see satisfying results following someone else's exercise/nutrition program. I just love seeing people achieve fitness goals, regardless of whose book or DVD they followed. I would be so happy if everyone could be in shape, because being happy with your own body goes way beyond just looks. Your mood improves dramatically, along with your energy level. You start becoming a more confident and positive person. People will be more attracted to the positive/confident energy you exude when being in shape.

Most people complain, think negatively and are unhappy with themselves. They choose to live that way instead of changing themselves. Why do they choose not to change for the better? Because they lack confidence. Confidence increases when goals are achieved, all types of goals: Short/long term, small/big, significant/insignificant, etc. People who lack confidence have a fear of failure. They have difficulty rebounding from failure and worry so much about what others think. That makes them want to avoid failure altogether, so as not to have other people think any less of them. Sad, isn't it? Of course it is. Confident and courageous people also have fear, but the difference is that they proceed forward despite the fear!

Think of a Spanish bullfighter, for example. All bullfighters are in fear when fighting the bull, but it doesn't stop them. Instead, fear is used as a motivation to train and prepare for the event. I was an All-American college wrestler, Golden Gloves boxer and mixed martial arts fighter. Let me tell you, before every match I was in fear. I knew that I had to proceed forward or else the feeling of guilt for not fighting would be far worse than losing the fight itself.

Another example is how many guys out there, myself included, who regret not asking out a certain woman because of fear of rejection. Many of us have had this experience, I'm sure! Well, I would much rather try asking her out and have her say no—and perhaps even throw her drink at my face—than to never have even tried! Am I right? I bet! Most people don't regret their failures nearly as much as regretting the chances they never took. Life is so short and youth is great, so why not extend our youth as long as possible? Sounds like a miracle? Perhaps, but it's possible through my system of healthy eating, exercise and rest. You can be strong, fit, healthy, positive, fearless, etc.

My system of nutrition/exercise differs greatly from others because I will commit to working with you for the long-term. This is crucial in order to reach your goals. Many changes in your eating and training will need to be made throughout the body-transforming process. Each and every individual has a completely different metabolism, lifestyle, taste in foods, training preference and most of all fitness goals. I will see to it that you will be custom-fitted with your own individualized meal plan and exercise regimen. We'll constantly make adjustments in order to achieve maximum results in the shortest amount of time possible.

I have read numerous fitness/diet books and I must say that many of them were a tremendous help. I definitely acquired a lot of knowledge reading them and I am grateful to the authors. However, all of the other books have one thing in common: When you are finished reading, you are now on your own. At the end of the book the last sentence always pretty much says "Good luck, you are on your own now." There is no aftercare, no individualization in workouts, diet, etc. It's as if you are just a number or a means of financial income. For me, the greatest reward would be the positive results you achieve from what you learn after reading this book. Getting in shape can really be a fantastic journey, especially if the journey is custom-made for you!

Chapter 8: All in a Day's Work

Maintaining a daily routine is a necessary step toward reaching your fitness goals. Is it easy? Not initially, but in the long run it is, because exercising and eating well-balanced meals takes dedication and discipline. This is so much easier than living with the guilt of being unhappy with your body, which leads to a lower quality of life! How? When you're unhappy with your body, you miss out on life. You avoid the beach, outdoor activities and get-togethers. Then your means of having fun becomes limited and more expensive, while being much less enjoyable. Out-of-shape people end up staying home more, going out to eat more, buying expensive gifts, cars, jewelry etc. People who are happy with their body love showing it off by going to the beach, barbeques, walks in the park, enjoying sports, visiting friends, family, etc. Not only do they feel better, they have more fun and their fun is more economical as well. Come on, how much does playing a game of tennis cost, compared to going out to a fine restaurant? And who do you think is having more fun? Who's enjoying himself more, the guy riding a bicycle without his shirt and getting a few flirty looks from the opposite sex, compared to that out-of-shape person waiting in traffic in a beautiful and very expensive Mercedes Benz sports car? Same answer! That person on the bicycle is loving life—and at rock-bottom prices, too! Sounds to me like a win-win situation for everyone!

Now let's see what a day using my methods looks like. You will see what it is like to live a day as an extremely healthy person.

Advanced Fitness Schedule

7 A.M. Wake up, 1 cup black coffee

7:30 A.M. 30-minute jog

8 A.M. Breakfast: 1 scoop whey protein isolate blended with 5 almonds, 1/3 cup oats, ½ banana

10:30 A.M. Snack: 1 cup nonfat Greek yogurt

1 P.M. Lunch: 1 can sardines with cucumber

3:30 P.M. Snack: 1 apple, 1 tablespoon all-natural peanut butter

5 p.m. snack: 1 scoop whey protein isolate blended with 5 walnuts, 1 apple

5: 30 P.M. 1 hour weight training or calisthenics

7 P.M. Dinner: 6 ounces London broil, steamed vegetables, 1 cup whole grain pasta

10 P.M. Snack if needed: 1 cup cooked egg whites

The advance version might seem like a tremendous sacrifice, but it really isn't—you never go hungry, for example, because you have lots of snacks. The rewards of using my methods far outweigh the sacrifices you make. As your body improves, they will seem well worth the commitment invested! You will look and feel better in every way! Confidence, attitude, complexion, appearance, sleep quality, energy level, patience, etc. will all improve! You will be amazed!

OK, I will admit that this advanced version may be a lot for most people's busy schedules. I will give you a beginner's and intermediate example of the perfect day to help you achieve the body you want!

Beginner's Fitness Schedule

8 A.M. Breakfast: 1 cup low-fat cottage cheese, black coffee or tea

10:30 A.M. Snack: 1 can or pouch of salmon, small salad

1 P.M. Lunch: grilled chicken sandwich on whole-grain bread

3:30 P.M. Snack: 1 cup nonfat Greek yogurt, 5 walnuts

5 P.M. Gym: 20 minutes treadmill, 5 sets pushups, 5 sets lat machine pull-downs, 5 sets free squats

6 P.M. Dinner: 5 ounces London broil, 1 sweet potato, 1 small green salad with oil and vinegar dressing

9 P.M. Snack if you are hungry: 5 ounces grilled turkey breast, steamed vegetables

Intermediate Fitness Schedule

7 A.M. black coffee or tea

7:30 A.M. 30 minutes house cleaning (light cardio)

8 A.M. Breakfast: 1 cup egg whites, 1 yolk, 1 fruit

10:30 A.M. Snack: 1 cup nonfat Greek yogurt with 5 almonds

1 P.M. Lunch: grilled chicken sandwich on whole-grain bread

3:30 P.M. Snack: 1 can light tuna in water, 1 tomato

5 P.M. Gym: 5 sets push-ups, 5 sets pull-ups

6 P.M. Dinner: 5 ounces broiled fish, 1 sweet potato, steamed broccoli

9 P.M. Snack if you are hungry: 1 cup egg whites, 1 fruit, 5 walnuts

These are three options, beginners, intermediate and advanced levels. All three will work well for you. To reach your maximum potential, however, many adjustments need to be frequently made to better suit you and to optimize your progress. Think of this as a lifestyle, with me as your assistant and coach. This is a joint effort between both of us. Together we will develop the body you have long desired. I am confident in my work because I have seen so much progress with my clients. Please feel comfortable and confident with my options, because achieving your fitness goals is closer than you could ever imagine!

Chapter 9: Reap the Benefits

Follow these simple methods and positive benefits will show—some immediately, others later on. There are virtually no negative drawbacks to this type of lifestyle. Most things have their drawbacks. A powerful car uses more fuel, a large beautiful house costs a lot of money, a motorcycle is easy to park but a nightmare to drive in the rain. But in the world of health and exercise, there are virtually no negatives, no drawbacks, none! You will look better, feel better, be healthier, have increased energy level, improved sleep, less stress, more confidence—and you'll save money in so many ways.

Healthy people are more productive, get sick less often, and require less money for entertainment, because going for a bike ride or swim is free. Overweight and unhealthy people cannot do this, which also leads them to more impulse spending, impulse eating, and other instant satisfactions. They're not happy with their appearance which leads to unhappiness, depression, spending more money for fun, doctor's visits, etc. A person in shape has more of a happy-go-lucky attitude. He or she is happier with their appearance. These people also benefit from the great feeling of endorphins, the brain chemicals that cause "runner's high," that are released while exercising. The only possible negative drawback could be the thirty minutes per day that's dedicated to exercising. That thirty minutes is an investment, because you will get so much more out of the remaining twenty three and a half hours in the day. You will be supercharged all day, which will enable you to accomplish more throughout the day and in a much happier way. Simply said, you will be more productive and in a much happier mood!

Exercise and dieting have definitely changed my life for the better. I'm not the only one, so I really want you to feel the great feeling that I feel. I want you to have the health benefits, and of course, looking better has its perks too! That's a winning proposition for everyone!

As you continue reading this book, you will notice which approach to getting into shape will work best for you. Once again my methods and approach toward getting into shape are quite different than most everyone else's in that fun is a top priority.

Having fun is extremely important because it will improve your quality of life and allow you to commit more to your progress. If you're having fun, you won't mind spending time at the gym and eating nothing but healthy foods. There's no doubt that fitness is a long-term affair, so enjoy it as much as you can, from the diet right down to the workouts. As a personal trainer I have witnessed many people get both into shape and unfortunately get out of shape as well. What I've learned from observing them is that it is extremely important to arrange different workouts and meal plans for each individual. This is called fitness customization. Every person has different tastes, fitness goals, lifestyle and genetics. Why not custom arrange specific workout routines and meal plans for each person? Training my clients with this principal quickly led to dramatically positive results. My clients noticed the changes, both physical and mental, almost immediately. Helping my clients make psychological improvements and have a better outlook on life is extremely important to me. This is another area where my approach towards getting into shape different from most everyone else's.

The bottom line is I really want you to get into shape, no matter what the obstacles are. Obstacles are just opportunities to reach new and higher levels.

Chapter 10: Keeping Fit While Away from Home

Even though health and fitness are my passion, there is still so much more for me to learn. In fact, it seems as if the more I learn, the more I realize that there is so much that I don't know.

Realizing this is a huge motivational factor toward my desire to educate myself on a constant basis. The truth is that there is no secret or shortcut to getting into shape. There may be many promises but few, if any results. And results are the true barometer that measures success.

Getting into shape doesn't begin with buying a gym membership or with vacation tickets that are two weeks away. Don't get me wrong—"crash course" weight loss is possible, but it certainly is not the best approach. It will hinder muscle growth and toning, and it can cause havoc on your health and quality of life, plus you're certain to gain back the weight and some extra as soon as you go off the diet. People want fast results, but what happens here is that people to either skip or ignore the process of getting into shape.

Obviously there are many processes we would like to skip. For example, we would much rather fly in a jet to Europe as opposed to a boat ride, because getting to Europe quickly is the goal. Most of the time, though, the process is overlooked. When this happens, we begin to race to achieve results. Rushing to do anything is a recipe for failure. Optimum results in everything require knowledge, preparation, desire and patience. So before you decide to join that gym or soccer team, understand that you must first make a serious commitment.

Understand that the results you want will not happen overnight. Some results, notably a better outlook on life, will happen quickly, but most people overlook that and want to see a better physique instead. The process of getting into shape doesn't happen overnight, so why not enjoy the journey? Think of how you look for a job. Most people try to find the highest-paying job, and then see what the job is and if they're qualified, right? Of course they do. But is that the best approach? What is our true wealth? Money or happiness? Happiness of course!

Success doesn't bring happiness but happiness will bring you success. Now let's again go job searching again, but this time let's look for a job that we can enjoy, where our passion is first, and then check to see the salary. To earn a lot of money at a job, chances are that you will need to be very good at whatever the job entails. We all know that to be good at something we have to apply a lot of dedication and time. When you love your job, you will be very dedicated and passionate about it. Spending long hours committing to your work won't seem like a burden at all. Eventually, you will end up making more money because you have become a master at your profession. In this way, you'll be twice as successful, because you will be making money and you will be happy because you are doing what you love.

Another great example is a professional athlete. When interviewed, none of them ever say that they wanted to follow some other profession but instead chose to be an athlete because the money was better. They chose their sport because they loved it. Most of them worked many years in the lower levels, being very dedicated but making little or no money, before they got that big contract. This is the perfect example of following your passion first. Whether your salary is small or large, you will already be wealthy in happiness.

How can my training methods be applied to getting into shape while traveling? You may surprised to learn that same formula can be applied anywhere you happen to be. That's because how we get into shape varies tremendously. The question to "What is the best way to get into shape?" is "The way you like." And if you like to travel, you can use that to get into shape.

By traveling, I don't mean going someplace else to lie on a couch watching TV and drinking a beer, nor simply sitting in a sauna or going to a music concert. Your travel needs to be active to maintain your training. It could include going to the beach and going for a jog or bike ride or even doing push-ups or pull-ups. To be more specific, the way you will get into shape can be custom-made for you depending on your preferred workout and diet options.

Let's think of going out to eat at a restaurant. After seating you at your table, the server will give you a menu and you choose the foods that you like from those on the menu. You're not going to ask for sushi at a Mexican restaurant, right? Now we can apply this to getting into shape. There are many workouts and healthy meal plans available on a "fitness menu" so the key is to chose the healthy food options that you like. Don't pick the ones that your friend used and got great results, because that plan may not work for you or you may not enjoy it, and vice versa.

Enjoy is another key word because we are always good at things we enjoy. Activities that usually sound like a drag, such as a job, a diet and an exercise program can be made into fun activities. For example, let's start with your cardio workout. Cardio means increasing your heart rate, so why don't you personally choose the activity that will do that? Often people choose a treadmill or a Stairmaster or an elliptical machine as their first choices for a cardio workout only because they feel that they have to, as opposed to want to. Now let's say that as a child you really enjoyed playing table tennis, basketball, bike riding, dancing, or whatever else. Doesn't it make sense to engage in an activity that you will enjoy and benefit from the cardio workout as well?

Let's now look at your resistance workout. Instead of lifting weights, you may enjoy calisthenics such as push-ups and pull-ups more, so why not do them? Along the same lines, let's talk about your diet. With so many healthy meal variations, there will be a few that you especially like, so why not choose those? If you're not crazy about egg whites, then eat fish, or turkey breast, or chicken breast, or even whey protein. If you really like oatmeal, then why would you eat sweet potatoes or brown rice? Oatmeal is a great food especially for you—because you like it! Do you see why enjoying everything in your fitness program is so important for happiness and success? When you're enjoying your training routines, meal plans and cardio workout, creating the body you want is so much easier. It's like you're breezing through it! This also means that you can continue to look great for a very long time, because you have the most enjoyable options available. Because you're having fun, you can stick with your program. Eating and training is now fun!

Chapter 11: Traveling the Healthy Way

Today we're all so busy that many of us don't have the time to eat well-balanced, home-cooked meals in the comfort of our own homes. We end up having to eat out a lot, from business meals at high- end restaurants to hotdog stands and everywhere in between. Usually dining out comes at a hefty price, not only in cost but in food quality and your body's health and appearance. All are losing propositions.

When we eat out, sometimes it's a luxury, such as a fancy restaurant dinner on a Saturday night. Enjoyable, but expensive and often with the drawback of excessive calories. More often, we're eating out during our lunch break on a typical workday. Less expensive than a fancy restaurant, but with the same calorie drawback. Sometimes we're eating out alone because we're traveling on business. You might be on an expense account, which makes the temptation of extra calories even harder to resist.

A lot of eating out will cause weight gain in the long run. Most people accept this. They know that eating out is not the healthiest option, but they like the convenience and enjoy the food. To a point, they are correct. My goal with this book is to show you how you can continue to enjoy eating out by adding a healthy "twist" to what you order. You'll be able to eat at any restaurant without weight gain or negative health consequences.

I know you're wondering if this is really possible. Of course it is! Not only is this possible, but it is possible within all financial budgets, demographics, even if you are a vegetarian. I decided to write this book because as a certified personal trainer I have helped many people achieve their fitness, appearance and health goals. During this process we needed to adjust their eating habits in numerous ways. Clients would often tell me, "Chris, I can't do this because I'm always on the road" or "Chris, I can't afford steamed salmon at a restaurant every day." Fortunately, I came up with solutions to all of my clients eating obstacles. Almost all were happy but a few were not, because some people look for excuses not to succeed! Crazy, isn't it? But it's true that some of us don't have the confidence to succeed, making failure the easier option. "Could of, would of, should of" is something we've all heard that many times. Let's not use these same old excuses. What do success and performance require? What is the key ingredient to success and happiness? Confidence! "Believe and you shall achieve!"

Success takes belief, but it also takes sufficient preparation. Why am I sounding like a coach instead of an author right now? Because the psychology of fitness is the structure to maintaining a healthy lifestyle. A building is built on a solid foundation, right? Well the same goes for you. You must have a solid foundation when living a healthy lifestyle. You must really want to lose weight and be fit. As a personal trainer I have seen people succeed and fail many times. So what's the difference? Determination. Let's face it, it's not that simple. I want you to be hungry, determined, and relentless, because that's how you will succeed.

So before we even start, I need you to be ready for a major change in your daily life and attitude—a change for the better! Let's build that solid foundation with confidence and determination and the rest is easy. Don't be in this just for the results, be in this for the process. It's a nice journey toward being in the best shape of your life. Let's enjoy the ride!

Chapter 12: Traveling in Shape

Traveling is an enjoyable part of many of our lives. Unfortunately, traveling also leads to breaking your routines. To most of us, breaking our routine means inconvenience—and inconvenience leads to uncomfortable situations that negatively impact our health and appearance. When we think of traveling we think of eating out, missing workouts and sleeping in uncomfortable beds. Even a local traveling salesperson who has the comfort of sleeping at home every night has the inconvenience of driving all day and dealing with traffic and other stressful situations. The traveler is also subject to fast food, restaurants, business lunches and alcohol consumption. Missing workouts often comes along with this hectic lifestyle. Whenever we break our routines, it seems as though chaos happens.

Breaking your healthy routine because of travel no longer needs to happen. I have created a series of exercises that require no machines or gym equipment. Simply by using your own body weight, you can exercise your entire body in 30 minutes or less. Never could I stress enough how important it is to exercise and keep your routine wherever you may be and regardless of the situation. I have been exercising my entire life and it has become a source of fulfillment and happiness. The days that I don't exercise, I feel a void. It almost seems as if the day will not feel complete nor 100 percent. I can't seem to live without that euphoric feeling that exercise provides. After a nice workout you have the feeling that any goal you may have is within reach! Who wouldn't want to experience that great feeling every day? Having regrets is a part of our lives but exercise will never be one of them. Many times I have literally dragged myself to my workout because the drive just wasn't there that day. As soon as the workout was halfway through my feelings started to improve. By the time the workout was over, I felt awesome! I was so glad to have worked out that my mood was elevated to the highest level!

That great euphoric post-workout feeling usually happens in this time frame: The first fifteen minutes I'm dragging myself. Between fifteen and thirty minutes, I begin feeling pleased that I am exercising instead of being lazy. After thirty minutes the endorphin high begins taking effect so now I start feeling that I am on top of the world! That endorphin high usually lasts up to a few hours after exercising.

You will succeed in getting into great shape when you look at exercising as not only a means to looking better but most of all to feeling better. Your mind will open up to new dimensions! After a thirty-minute workout, the remaining twenty three and a half hours in the day will be so much better! Trust me! You will feel more alive, confident, tighter, and more patient. You will sleep better and have a happier demeanor. Whatever you engage in after your workout is at least 100 times better in every way. Guaranteed! Being in shape is simply a win-win situation whichever way you look at it.

In all my years of training never have I heard anyone who was in shape regret being fit. Even if you can not seem to make your way to a gym due to traveling for work or vacation, I have a proven, simple method to either make you fit or maintain your shape. You will not believe how easy to be fit it really is!

Chapter 13: Eat Right While Traveling (Advanced Version)

Being away from the luxury of your home kitchen makes it more difficult to watch what you eat. While you're traveling, restaurants play a large part in your life. Choosing the healthiest restaurants and meals is of the utmost importance. Cooking healthy meals at home to pack up and take with you is the healthiest option of all, but often this is not possible due to time restraints or other factors. Drinking at least 2 quarts daily is important for enabling the body to function at its best. Try to drink only water with an occasional coffee or tea but beware that caffeine will dehydrate your body so make sure to drink plenty of water.

Restaurants are everywhere, as are food stands and delis. These places can be healthy choices, but that depends completely on what you order. Because I'm always out and about myself, eating on the road is part of my lifestyle, so I know it can be hard to make good choices. Between my nutrition education and a lot of trial and error, I've learned how to narrow down the healthier meal options no matter what type of food establishment you are eating in. Whether you're eating fast food or in a five-star restaurant, you can still maintain a great body.

Best Fast Food Choices

McDonald's
McGrill chicken breast sandwiches; don't eat the bread

Garden salad with low-calorie dressing (avoid added cheese or croutons)Burger King
Grilled fish sandwich (don't eat the bread)
Garden salad with low-calorie dressing

Wendy's
Fish sandwich without the bun
Garden salad with jalapeño peppers, low-calorie dressing

KFC
Chicken breast without the skin
Steamed vegetables

Boston Market
Turkey breast or chicken breast without the skin
Steamed vegetables or green salad

Street Vendors
Gyro with chicken without the yogurt sauce
Chicken and vegetable souvlaki

Sports Stadium
Hot dog without the bun
Small bag of pretzels

Pizza Places
Scungili salad
Grilled chicken breast with broccoli rabe
Grilled chicken breast with greens, small portion plain pasta

Taco Stand
Chicken taco with no cheese or sauce and plenty of greens

Movie Theater
Popcorn without butter

Diners
Broiled fish
Salad with lettuce, cucumber, tomato, olive oil and vinegar dressing
Grilled chicken breast
Steamed vegetables
Greek salad
London broil
Steamed vegetables
Hard-boiled egg whites
Egg white and vegetable omelet
Low-fat cottage cheese with fresh fruit

Fast Casual Restaurants (Applebee's, Houlihan's, etc.)
Grilled fish
Steamed vegetables
London broil
Salad with low-calorie dressing
Steamed vegetables mixed with plain pasta and salad

Chinese Restaurants
Steamed shrimp and vegetables with rice
Steamed chicken and vegetables with rice (brown rice if available

Japanese Restaurants
Sashimi
Salad
Seafood in pot of hot water
Brown rice sushi
Hibachi steak with vegetables
Hibachi chicken with vegetables

Seaweed salad
Italian Restaurants
Shrimp cocktail
Salad
Grilled fish with steamed vegetables
Portobello mushrooms
Broiled chicken breast
Clams on the half shell
Fish with broccoli rabe and olive oil

Spanish Restaurants
Clams on the half shell
Salad with oil and vinegar dressing
Broiled seafood with steamed vegetables
Steamed mussels with lemon
Steamed lobster
Steamed broccoli
Octopus in vinaigrette or olive oil
Grilled chicken breast
Steamed vegetables

Thai Restaurants
Steamed fish
Green salad
Steamed shrimp dumplings

Greek Restaurants
Grilled octopus
Green salad
Grilled seafood with lemon and olive oil
Cucumber, olive and tomato salad
Grilled whole fish
Seafood salad

Chicken breast with olive oil and lemon
Greek salad
Grilled calamari

Indian Restaurants
Green salad
Chicken tandoori

South American Restaurants
Shrimp ceviche
Green salad
Broiled fish with vegetables
Octopus ceviche
Chicken breast grilled with lime

Brazilian Restaurants
Chicken breast skewers
Green salad
Salmon and vegetables skewers

Mexican Restaurants
Guacamole salad
Spicy grilled fish
Grilled chicken breast with onions

Polish Restaurants
Red cabbage salad
Boiled beef
Cucumber and dill salad
Boiled chicken with sauerkraut

Russian Restaurants
Smoked herring

Low-fat kefir (yogurt)
Pickled cabbage
Boiled beets
Pickled sturgeon

What to Drink

A reminder about what to drink: Always have plenty of plain water with every meal. If you wish, have one glass of red or white wine with dinner. Diet sodas or unsweetened iced tea are also good choices.

As you can see, healthy dining can pretty much be accomplished anywhere. With just that little bit of know-how, going to a restaurant while maintaining that great body will be a breeze. Next you will learn how to put this all together, making it simple for you to follow.

It is important to know that meal timing is very important. Try to eat small meals every two to four hours. Eating small meals frequently helps keep your metabolism elevated which means your body consumes more overall calories throughout the day. Eating in this manner also keeps your body's digestive system working efficiently throughout the entire day. Efficient food digestion equals more energy across the day. With smaller meals, you don't experience the insulin spike from eating fast-acting carbohydrates. An insulin spike leads to feeling tired and hungry after eating and in the long-term leads to type two diabetes.

Eating a diet that is rich in protein, healthy fats and fiber will give you the great body you want and the energy you will need to live a healthier, happier and a more productive lifestyle—guaranteed! I will see to it that anywhere and at any time, regardless of your budget and time constraints, eating out will be a healthy, positive experience.

There is no reason why dining out should give you unwanted calories and hinder your progress toward having the body of your dreams. Remember that traveling and keeping a nice physique can go hand in hand. Many times in the past, I have felt sluggish and bloated because of eating the wrong foods while away from home. What an uncomfortable feeling that was! During the day, I am always out, which means eating out as well. Through trial and error and education I have learned to narrow my choices down to what works and what doesn't. A simple way is great, but a simple and fun way is even better. What I mean by this is that it must not only be effective but fun too. You have to be committed, so why not be committed to a more enjoyable workout and meal plan? There are many different ways that you can get into shape and many work quite well. People more knowledgeable than me abound, but what makes me different is my obsession with helping the people I work with achieve results and really enjoy their fitness and diet programs. Results are how progress and commitment are measured. Long-term commitment is much easier when you enjoy what you are doing. Yes, the process of getting into shape can be a lot of fun—it really can. Take it from me, the original "good time Charlie" himself!

Chapter 14: A Day on the Road!

Eating right is definitely an important step toward having a great body. Eating healthy food is necessary to build a great body, but just as important is how and when you eat. Proper food prepared the wrong way will hinder your progress toward getting into shape.

What does the "wrong way" actually mean?
1. Food portions which are either too big or too small.
2. Improperly balanced meals. For example, a meal with too many carbs and not enough protein; or with too much protein and not enough fat; or even too much fat and not enough protein or carbohydrates.
3. Eating at the wrong times, either too frequently or too sparingly.

Managing your food intake is extremely important. Knowing which foods to eat and when to eat them will play a tremendous part in achieving that lean and toned body you are looking for. Let's just say you went to the supermarket and bought all the right foods—chicken breast, egg whites, oatmeal, vegetables and fruit. With all of these great foods you are probably thinking, how could I go wrong? Easily. If your breakfast consists of egg whites and chicken breast, that's not a balance meal—it's all protein. Instead, have egg whites and oatmeal. The egg whites are the protein and oatmeal is the complex carbohydrate. Another improper would be having some steamed vegetables and oatmeal for lunch instead of the more balanced chicken breast and a sweet potato. The sweet potato is a complex carbohydrate and chicken is protein. Do you understand now how important it is to structure your meals properly?

Now let's say that instead of eating every two to four hours, you skipped breakfast and lunch but ate a triple-sized meal at dinner. You'd feel very bloated and tired afterward. Plus, because you didn't eat regularly during the day, you'll be starving by dinnertime. That means you're more likely to cheat on your diet.

Having the right food, preparing it the right way and eating regularly cannot be overlooked. You do have to plan carefully. Imagine going on a vacation without planning. Not a good idea at all. Even if your vacation destination is really nice, everything else would be a mess, from the overbooked hotel to going at the wrong time, like hurricane season. A nice vacation can be ruined by lack of planning. The same goes for food. You can buy the healthiest food, but your body will not benefit unless the meals are properly prepared and eaten at the right times.

Exactly when and what to eat is different for everyone. Some healthy foods work better than others for different people. In time, you will begin to choose the healthy foods you enjoy eating and get know the best times throughout the day for you to eat. This is called "meal customization" and it works very effectively. When I first began eating well-balanced meals to improve my physique, I was kind of doing it the hard way. I made a lot of typical mistakes.

The hard way means only eating the meals that were recommended to you by someone else. Even if that person had great results on himself eating those same meals, they might not work well for you. I was always asking people with great bodies questions on what they ate and I studied nutrition quite a bit as well. I was trying to find the best foods for me to make dieting a lot more pleasant. For a while, I was just eating the foods that I thought would provide the best results possible. I felt miserable and bored with those foods, which always led to me quitting that particular diet. After a while, I realized that I needed to come up with fun ways to eat healthy foods. Of the healthy meal options, I now began carefully choosing the foods that were the most enjoyable for me to eat. For example, instead of oatmeal I ate brown rice, instead of broccoli I ate cucumbers, instead of salmon I ate herring, etc. By eating this way, all of a sudden my quality of life improved. I was happier and eager to proceed with the diet, and also I had fewer junk food cravings. Eating healthy to achieve a great body was now so much easier. That made me able to be more committed to the long-term, which in the past I couldn't do.

Success in improving your body comes after commitment and dedication. That will be much easier once you narrow down which foods and workouts suit you best. Having the most fun possible while developing your body will totally ease the process.

Every person's day varies, so I'll give you a few examples of what and when to eat on an average day. Once again, these are merely examples—so many more meal options are available. Remember that the key to success here is keeping up a steady pace that you can continue. Have you ever seen a marathon runner sprinting at the beginning of the race? Of course not!

A Day on the Road

Breakfast
At a diner:
Egg white omelet (1 cup egg whites)
1 cup plain oatmeal
Coffee or tea with skim milk, zero-calorie sweetener

Mid-morning Snack (2 to 3 hours after breakfast)
1 apple

Lunch at Chinese Restaurant
Steamed shrimp with vegetables

Mid-Afternoon Snack (2 to 3 hours after lunch)
2 ounces (1 packet) almonds

Dinner at Italian Restaurant
Clams on the half shell
Broiled salmon with capers
Salad
Steamed vegetables

Another Day on the Go

Breakfast at IHOP
Egg Beater omelet
1 cup grits
Coffee or tea with skim milk, zero-calorie sweetener

Mid-Morning Snack (2 to 3 hours after breakfast)
1 cup nonfat Greek yogurt

Lunch at a Street Vendor
1 chicken gyro (no sauce)

Mid-Afternoon Snack (2 to 3 hours after lunch)
1 banana

Dinner at a Spanish Restaurant
Shrimp cocktail
Broiled red snapper with garlic
Salad
Steamed vegetables

Inexpensive Day on the Go

Breakfast at a deli
4 hard-boiled eggs (don't eat the yolks)

Mid-Morning Snack (2 to 3 hours after breakfast)
1 fruit

Lunch at a deli
Low-sodium chicken breast sandwich on whole-wheat bread with lettuce, tomato and mustard

Mid-Afternoon Snack (2 to 3 hours after lunch)
4 plain rice cakes

Dinner at a bagel shop
Egg whites on a plain bagel

There are many more meal options for you to choose from that will make your body transforming process as enjoyable as possible. Dieting, looking good, feeling great, can all be accomplished in a fun way, trust me. This is 100 percent true! We just need to find the meal combinations that are tailor-made for you. This is like clothing. What fits better? Clothing off the rack or clothing custom-tailored for you? Custom-tailored, of course! It's the same with a meal plan. I can custom-design it for you so you can breeze right through to get you the body you want quickly and enjoyably! Different restaurants, different countries—healthy meals are available everywhere.

It is now up to you to really want to take this to the next level. Never, ever forget that having the body you always wanted is within your grasp. Never is it too late or unattainable. Your destiny depends on the choices and preparations, as well as the sacrifices you make today. Every move you make should be toward improving the future. Remember that great accomplishments require dedicated preparation and perseverance. Never let setbacks or failures stop you. Instead, use them for experience and education. All dreams are possible and without any expiration dates. Go after it now, because life really is short and great health is priceless!

Chapter 15: On Your Way to Becoming a Better You

Is there an easier and faster way to eating healthy? Possibly, but now we talking about customizing your meal plan specifically for you. There is a lot to be said for meal customization. This is really taking your health, performance and appearance to the next level. It would be a lot easier for me to simply sell my books and just wish you the best, but my conscience will not allow this. Why not? Because my idea of success is happiness, and for me the ultimate happiness is seeing results with the people I work with in fitness. Fitness is my life, my passion, all day, every day. Nutrition, training and helping people are always on my mind. I'm always seeking new training and diet techniques I can use to make improvements in my own regimen and for my clients. Seeing my clients happier, leaner, stronger is such a personal joy and satisfaction for me. Writing this book, the first of more to come, is the first step in passing on my knowledge to help you reach your fitness goals. To further assist you as a traveler, I will soon have on the market the Everywhere Gym. I created this portable gym, weighing merely three pounds, for easy transport while you're traveling. It provide up to 80 pounds of cable resistance for a complete body workout. Small, lightweight and portable, it's perfect for training on the go.

The next few chapters will be devoted to teaching you how to work out when you are traveling or on the go and can't get to the gym. The upcoming chapters will be filled with exercises, using Chris's Everywhere Gym or full-body callisthenic exercises that are performed with only your own body weight—no gym equipment required. The next part of this book will show you, the busy traveler, how to take your physique to the next level through effective exercise routines.

Chapter 16: Exercising While on the Road

In the first part of the book we learned how to properly eat toward building a great physique even if you are always on the go. I will guarantee that by following my methods of effective eating and exercise, your life on the road will be more fulfilling, energetic, enjoyable and productive! Why not look fantastic everywhere that you go? Having a lean body and a glowing complexion will only add to your life and experiences. No longer will you need to be like the typical traveler, who feels and looks tired, run-down, irritable, impatient, bloated, and out-of-shape. Looking sloppy has never been in style, while the appearance of someone who takes care of himself will always command respect and positive attention. Be excited to travel, but be even more excited to go to these places looking fit, sharp and confident. Carrying a nice physique will guarantee the entire experience will be 100 percent better! Wait until you read the rest of this book, which focuses on workout routines, because you will experience more progress and improvements on your body. What an unbelievable feeling that is! Noticing steady improvement is something we strive for, achieving small goals little by little. The process will be fun! Let's enjoy it and move forward by learning effective on the road exercise routines!

In this and the following chapter I will teach you effective exercise routines that can be performed anywhere and in any type of environment. These routines are quick and simple. Throughout my many years of traveling and being on the road, I have really narrowed down the exercises that work. Bear in mind that some exercises work more effectively for some people. No two people are alike, so an exercise that works for one person may not work for the next. People also have preferences as to which exercises they enjoy doing. For example, someone achieves great results performing two different exercises, such as dips and push-ups, but really enjoys performing dips more than push-ups. Then why not just do push-ups to make the workout more enjoyable? The more enjoyable the workout, the more you will stick to it for the long run. Consistency is the key. To remain consistent, you must enjoy what you are doing. Throughout the years as a personal trainer I have witnessed people come and go. Boredom was their number- one reason for quitting. This is why I began the quest to change boredom into fun. My attention span has always been terrible. That hurt me in many ways, so I came up with a solution—variety. If you constantly change your workout and diet, chances are you will have more success. You will never be bored by a workout. You can prioritize workout with the exercised that are most enjoyable for you to perform. OK, working out may not be as much fun as going on a cruise through the Mediterranean, but keep in mind that you will enjoy that cruise a lot more if you are happy with the way your body looks. If you want your body to look its best, then working out is a must.

Now we have to chose the exercises that are the most fun for you while still being effective. Your body has muscles from top to bottom, so it's important to know which exercises will develop which muscles.

Chapter 17: Exercises for Away from Home

These are the names of the most effective exercises that you will need to perform in order to achieve or maintain the perfect body. You can see photos of them starting on page 00.

Chest
Push-ups
Dips
Isometric flyers

Back
Pull-ups

Legs
Free squats
Single leg squats
Romanian squats
Lunges
Hamstring curls

Shoulders
Arm spins
Inverted push-ups
Indian push-ups

Triceps
Push-downs
Diamond push-ups
Biceps
Isometric curls
Chin-ups

Abs
Sit-ups
Crunches
Leg raises

Chapter 18: Exercise Routines

In this chapter I will explain how to exercise each body part with different variations. The different variations are to further your choices of exercises, which will enable you to choose which is best for you. There are many effective workout routines, so you must choose the one that makes you most comfortable. When exercising, the number of sets and repetitions can change, according to your level of fitness and how you want your body to look. I give beginner, intermediate and advanced routines. Choose the right routine based on which category you are in.

Beginner Workout Routines

Chest and Triceps
Push-ups, hands wide apart: 5 sets, 10 reps

Back and Biceps
Pull-ups, wide grip: 5 sets, 7 reps

Thighs and Hamstrings
Free squats: 4 sets, 20 reps

Abs
Crunches: 50 reps

Intermediate Workout Routines

Chest and Triceps
Push-ups, hands shoulder-width apart: 4 sets, 15 reps
Dips: 4 sets, 12 reps

Back and Biceps
Pull-ups, wide grip: 4 sets, 10 reps
Chin-ups, palms facing you: 4 sets, 10 reps

Thighs and Hamstrings
Free squats: 4 sets, 25 reps
Lunges: 4 sets, 25 yards

Shoulders
Hand stand press: 3 sets, 10 reps
Indian push-ups: 3 sets, 10 reps

Abs
Crunches: 50 reps
Leg raises: 50 reps

Advanced Workout Routines

Chest
Push-ups, hands shoulder-width apart: 7 sets, 20 reps
Dips: 7 sets, 15 reps

Triceps
Push-downs: 4 sets, 25 reps
Diamond push-ups: 4 sets, 15 reps

Back
Pull-ups, wide grip: 7 sets, 12 reps
Pull-ups, close grip: 7 sets, 12 reps

Shoulders
Hand stand push-ups: 3 sets, 12 reps
Indian push-ups: 3 sets, 12 reps
Inverted push-ups: 3 sets, 12 reps

Biceps
Chin-ups, close grip: 4 sets, 10 reps
Isometric curls: 4 sets, 12 reps

Abs
Crunches: 100 reps
Sit-ups: 100 reps

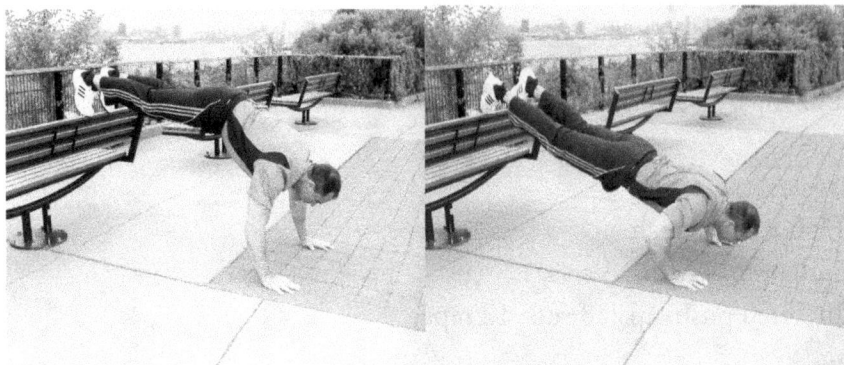

Push-Ups

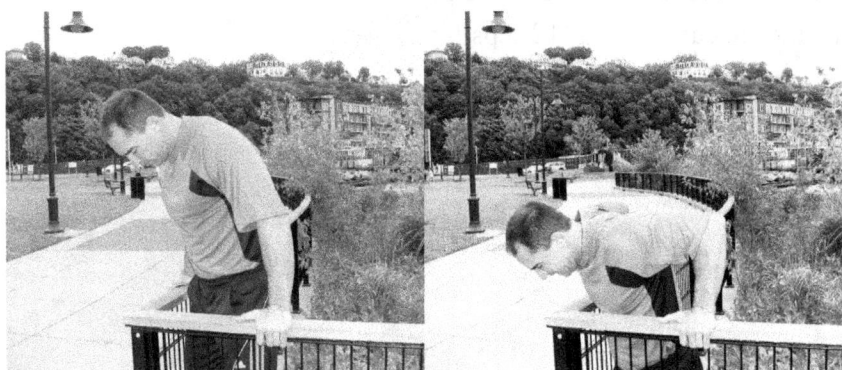

Dips

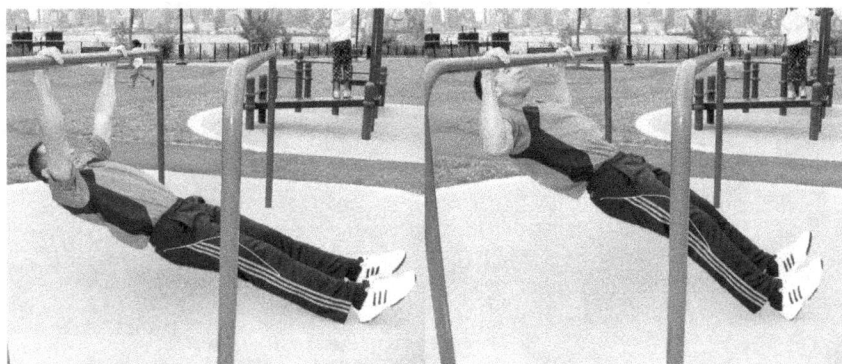

Back Rows

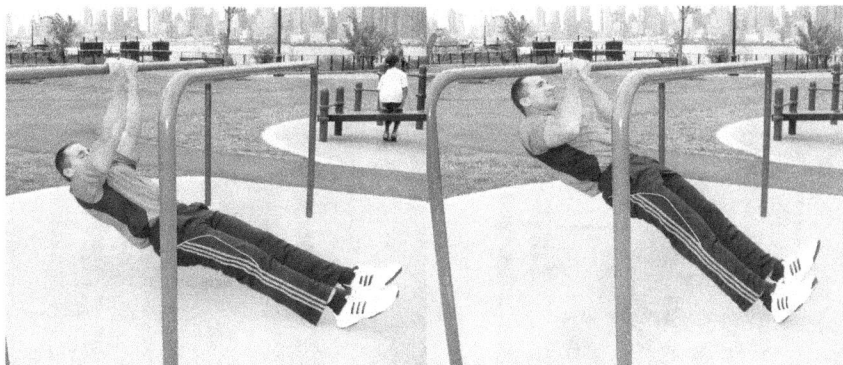

Back Rows (palms facing you)

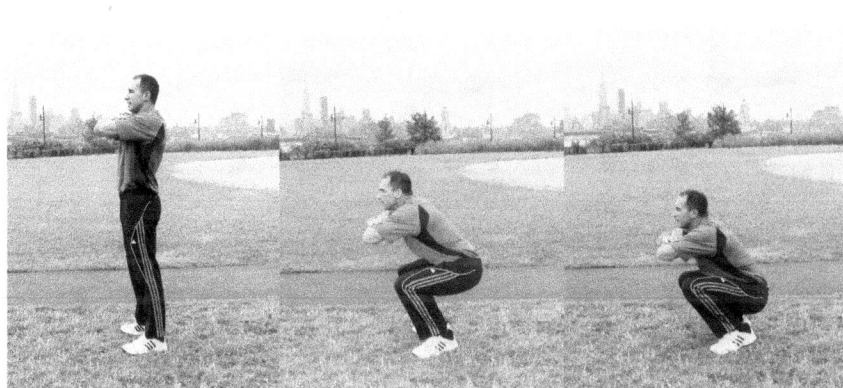

Free Squats

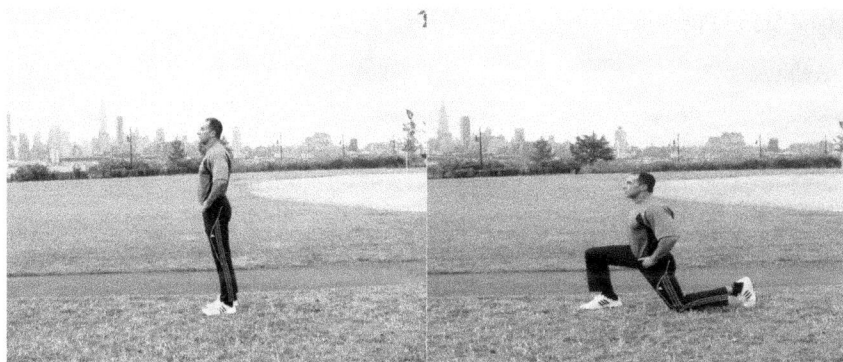

Walking Lunges

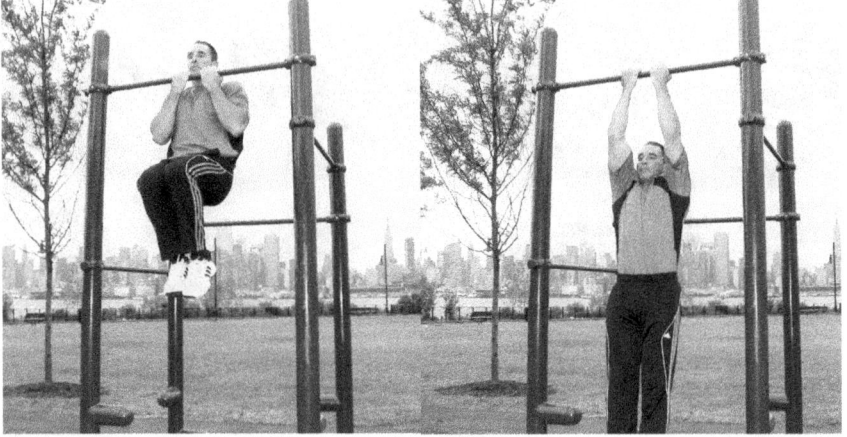

Chin-ups

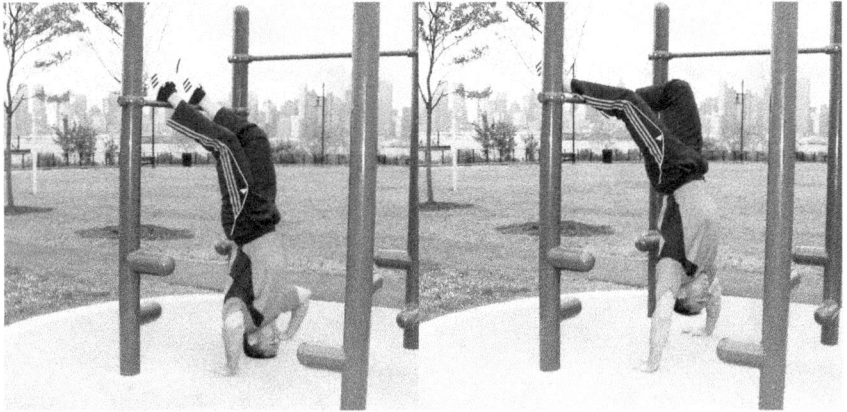

Hand Stand Push-ups

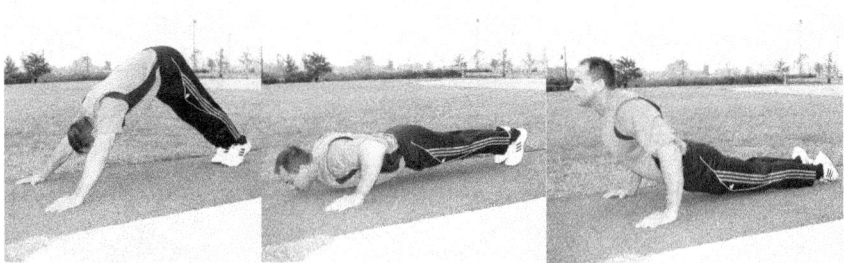

Indian Push-ups

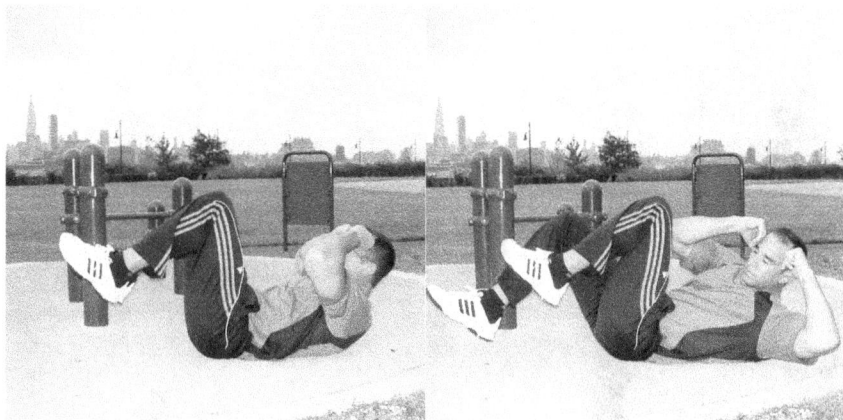

Bicycle Crunches

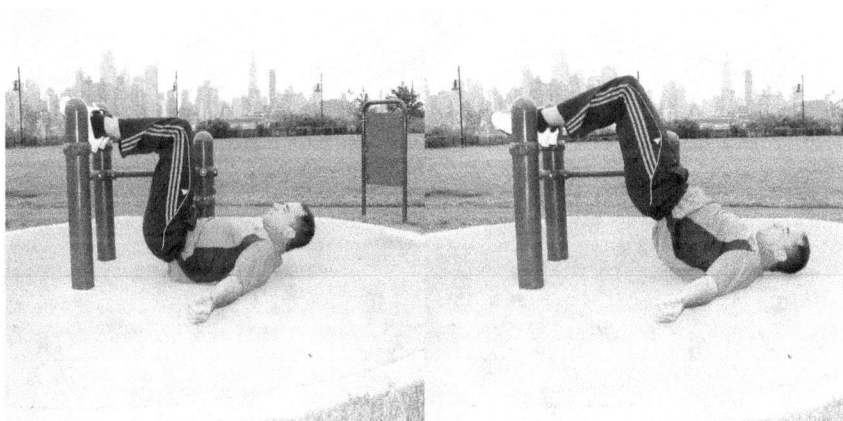

Hamstring Curls

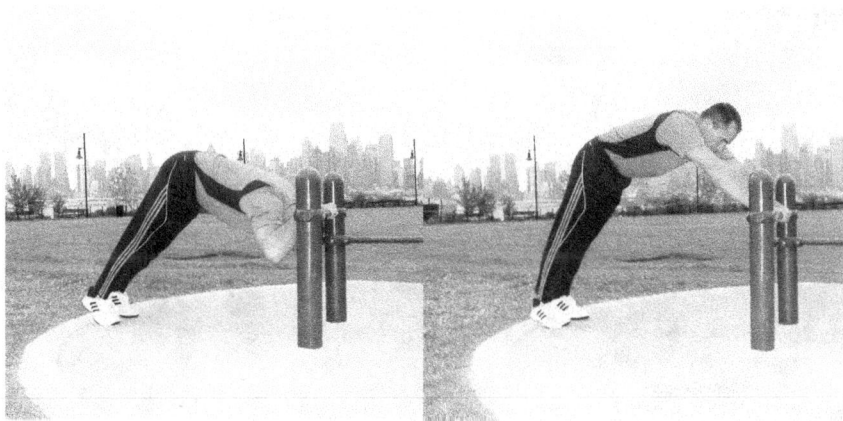

Triceps Push-down

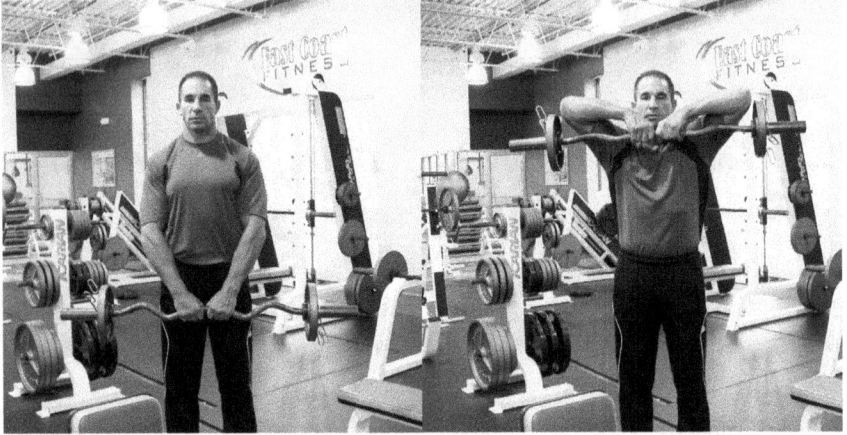

Upright Row

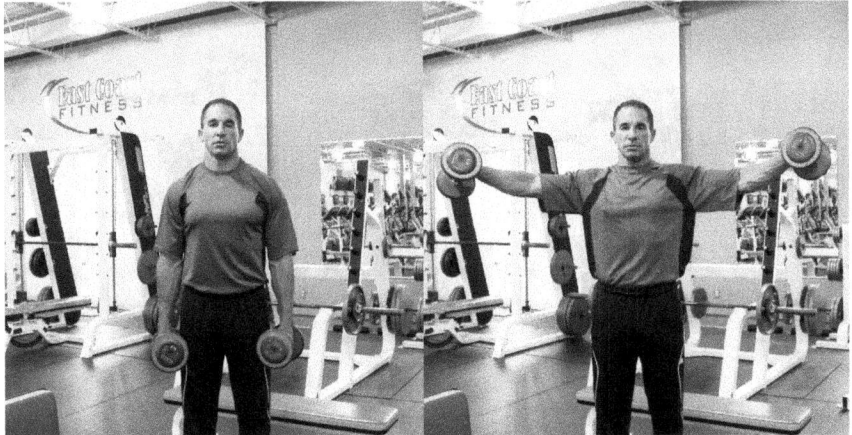

Lateral Raises

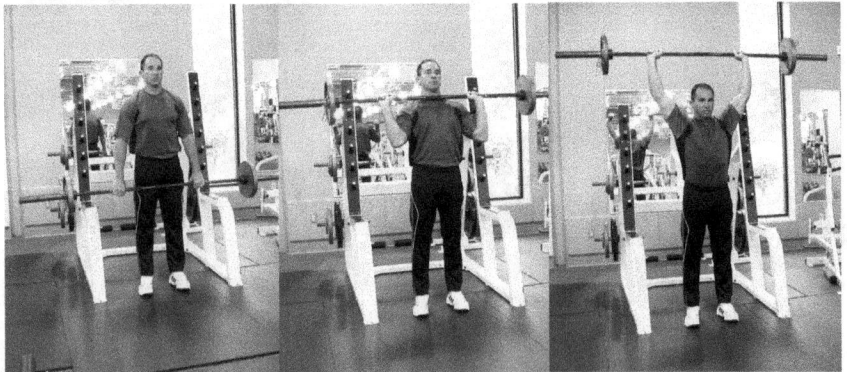

Compound Shoulder Press

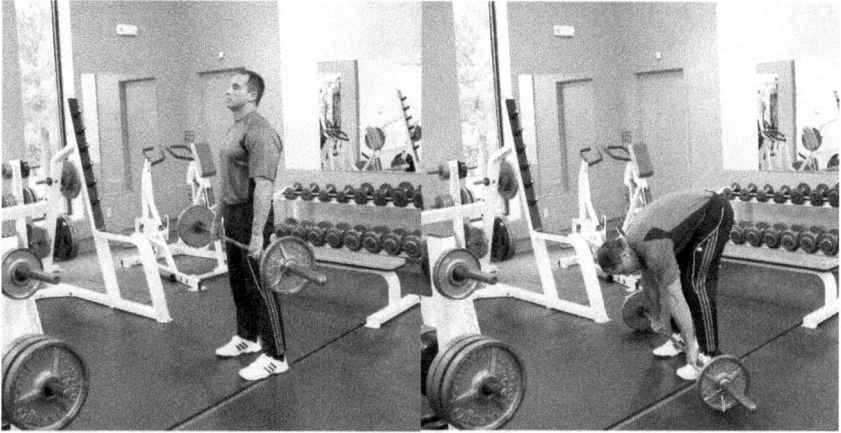

Stiff-leg Dead Lifts

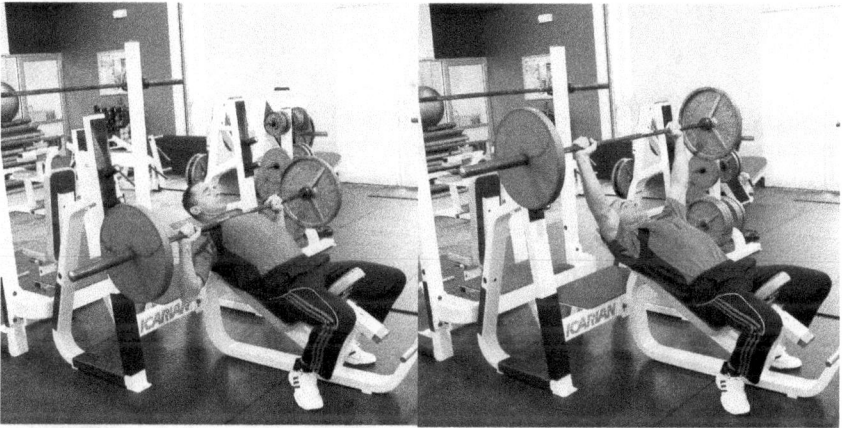

Incline Press

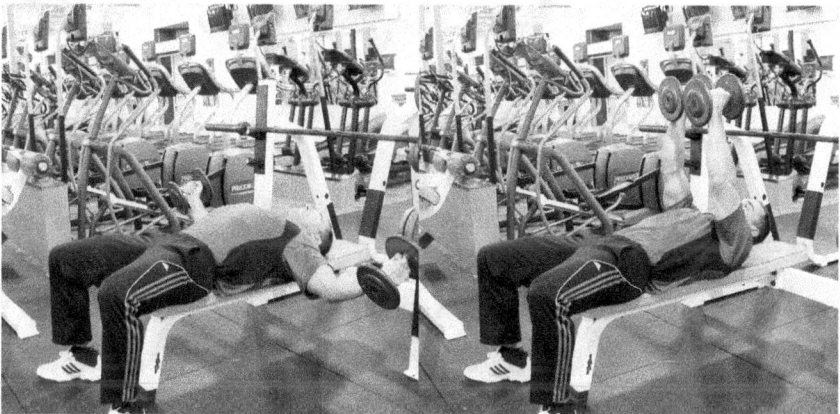

Flat Bench Flies

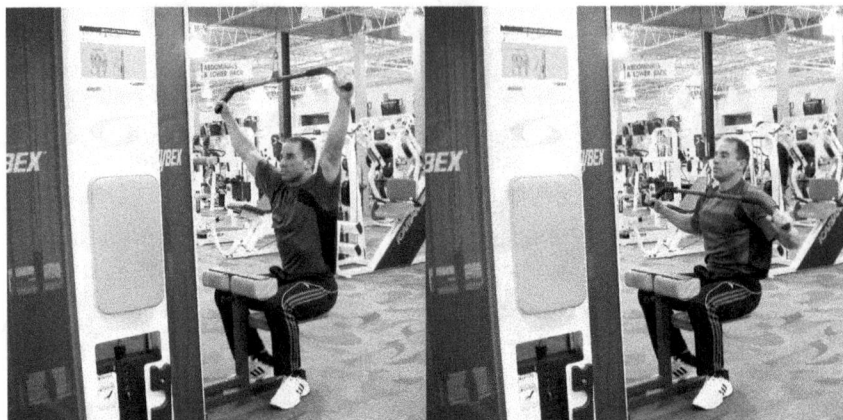

Lat Machine Pull-Downs

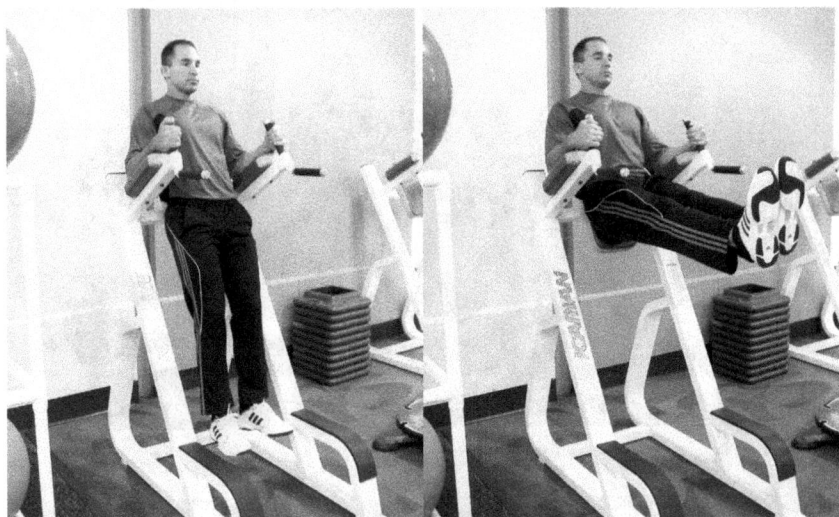

Leg Raises

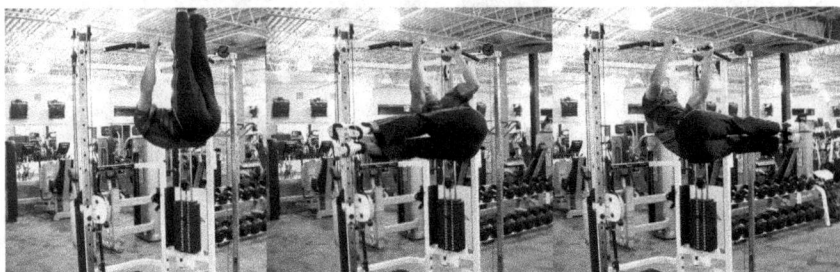

Windshield Wipers

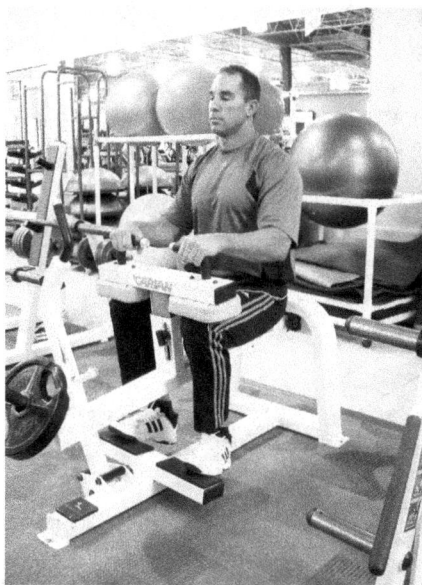

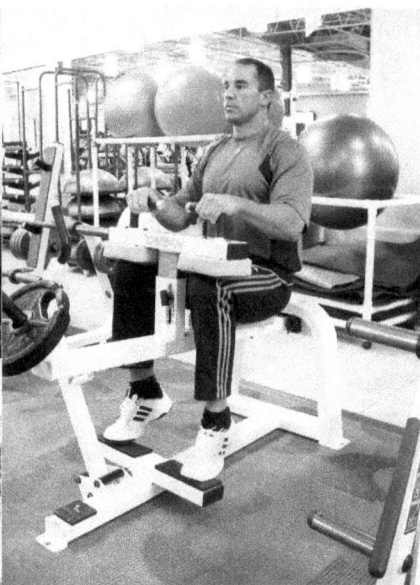

Seated Calf Raises

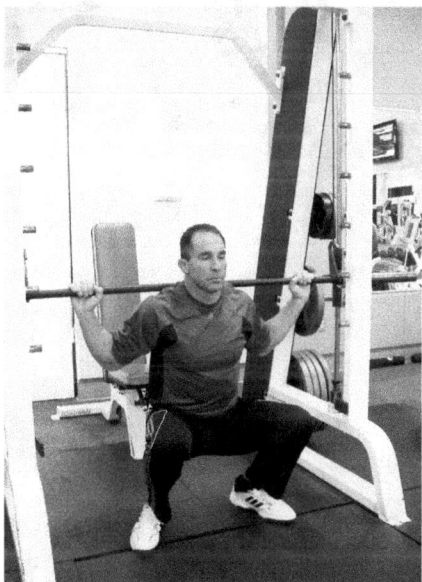

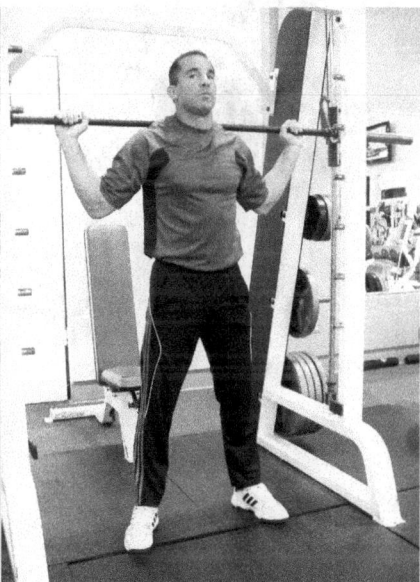

Smith Machine Squats

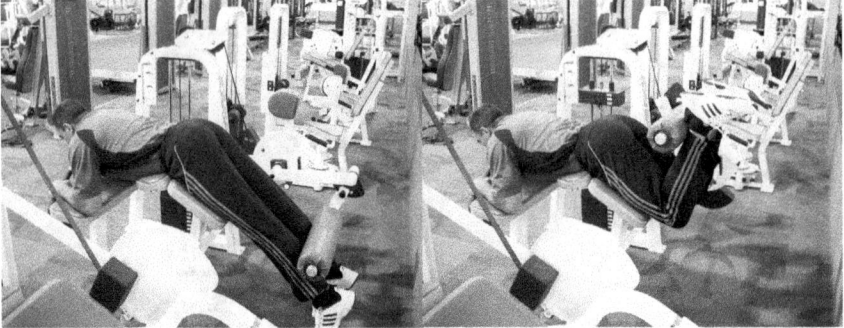

Leg Curls

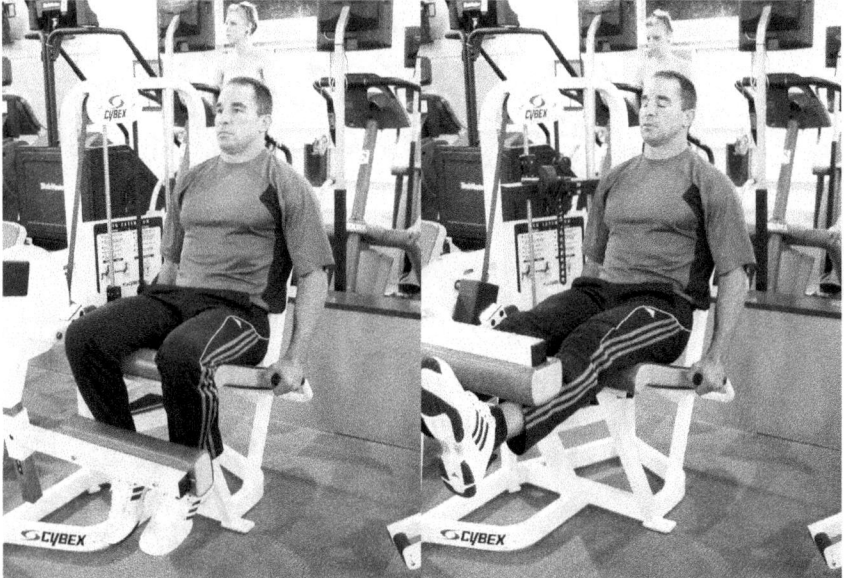

Leg Extensions

Chapter 19: A Week on the Go

Now I will teach you how you can properly train to maximize your progress while you are traveling away from your home and/or gym. Daily and weekly workout routines will be provided in order to keep your body fit, motivated and mentally charged all day and every day. A nice workout improves your body and mind. Your body and mind will become sharper as times goes on.

Beginner

Monday: triceps, chest, abs
Push-ups, hands close together: 5 sets, 10 reps
Push-ups, hands wide apart: 5 sets, 10 reps
50 crunches

Tuesday: legs, calves, back
Squats: 5 sets, 15 reps
Standing calf raises: 5 sets, 20 reps (super-set with squats)
Pull-ups: 7 sets, 8 reps

Wednesday
40-minute walk, jog or bicycle ride
Thursday: chest, triceps, abs, back
Dips: 7 sets, 8 reps
Chin-ups (palms facing you): 7 sets, 8 reps
Sit-ups: 50 reps

Friday: legs, hamstrings, calves
Walking lunges: 5 sets, 20 yards
Standing calf raises: 5 sets, 20 reps (super-set with lunges)

Saturday
Off

Sunday
Off

There we have a complete week of exercise for the beginner. It's a great idea to exercise every day. You feel more energized and in a better mood from the endorphins that are released when working out.

Intermediate

Monday: chest, triceps, abs
Push-ups: 5 sets, 12 reps
Dips: 5 sets, 12 reps
Crunches: 75 reps

Tuesday: back, biceps, calves
Chin-ups (palms facing you): 5 sets, 10 reps
Pull-ups, wide grip: 5 sets, 10 reps
Standing calf raises: 3 sets, 25 reps

Wednesday: legs, abs
Squats: 4 sets, 20 reps
Lunges: 4 sets, 20 yards
50 sit-ups

Thursday: shoulders, calves
Hand stand push-ups: 3 sets, 6 reps
Indian push-ups: 4 sets, 10 reps
Standing calf raises: 5 sets, 25 reps

Friday: back, biceps, chest, triceps
Chin-ups: 4 sets, 12 reps
Dips: 4 sets, 12 reps (super-set with chin-ups)
Push-ups: 4 sets, 12 reps
Pull-ups: 4 sets, 12 reps (super-set with push-ups)

Super-setting will also provide you a cardiovascular workout. I truly believe in super-setting and minimal rest time between sets. This will improve your cardiovascular system and also shorten the workouts. The intermediate athlete is already an extremely committed individual, so these workouts will benefit you to the fullest. You will really notice a better body and mental state of mind. From exercising so often, my mood is always elevated to the point where I don't even notice, because it's always like that. People often say I am a happy-go-lucky type of person due to my upbeat mood from exercising. Exercise is not just means to improve your body—it's a means to improve your mood as well.

Advanced (extreme fitness level)

Monday and Thursday: chest, triceps, back, biceps, abs
Pull-ups: 6 sets, 12 reps
Dips: 6 sets, 12 reps (super-set with pull-ups)
Chin-ups: 6 sets, 15 reps
Push-ups: 6 sets, 15 reps (super-set with chin-ups)
Isometric curls with triceps push-downs: 3 sets
Crunches: 50 reps
Sit-ups: 50 reps

Wednesday
1 hour jog, bicycle ride, play sports
Tuesday and Friday: shoulders, legs, calves
Hand stand push-ups: 5 sets, 10 reps
Indian push-ups: 5 sets, 12 reps
Squats : 5 sets, 25 reps
Lunges: 5 sets, 20 yards
Hamstring body curl: 5 sets, 15 reps
Standing calf raises: 5 sets, 30 reps

The advanced workout may seem difficult and lengthy, but don't be discouraged. You can still complete this workout in less than 30 minutes, although this will depend on your condition.

These exercise routines are only small taste of many possibilities. I can customize your workouts to further enhance your level of fitness. Customizing exercise routines for you personally will help you achieve that lean body that you are looking for.

Have you ever heard a wealthy person complaining about being too rich? Of course not! The same applies to fitness. Never have I heard any of my clients or anyone else in shape complain that they were in too good shape! It's never enough! That's the beauty of training. Improving your health and body has no plateau—you can keep improving always.

A good body is something everybody wants and money cannot buy. Only hard work, time and discipline will earn you a great physique. Remember, styles and fads come and go, here today, gone tomorrow. Whether it's clothing, perfume, tattoos, piercings, hairstyles, etc., a toned, in-shape body is always in style—back then, now, and in the future. When you are in shape, your clothing will look better on you, your complexion will improve and so will your mood and confidence. Having a fit body leads you to a chain reaction of many positive things that will make life better. Most of all enjoy the workouts, the dieting, and the process toward reaching your fitness goals. It is a wonderful experience and journey!

Enjoy the ride that I am about to send you on! As a person who's been training and in shape for my entire life, I've learned many techniques on nutrition and training over the years. Every year, I would always try to acquire more knowledge to help get me into shape easier and faster. At first, the workouts and dieting were extremely difficult and no fun at all. Why? Because they weren't custom-made for me. Little did I know that if my workouts and meal plans were adjusted, my transition into getting into shape would be that much easier. When I finally discovered this, what a tremendous break that was! No longer would I not like the foods I was eating or the workouts I was doing.. This didn't happen overnight, but the wait was definitely worth it. The time spent on dieting and training seemed to fly by. Have you ever heard the term "time flies when you're having fun?" This is the exact message I am trying to relay to you! Eating right and exercising can be very enjoyable because you are the boss, meaning that only you choose your workouts and meal variations. Sounds great, right? Well, there is a catch. You can't choose any workout or any meal plan. For example, video games don't count as working out and eating cupcakes or junk food doesn't count as a good meal plan. When eating, try to think of food as refueling your body with high-octane jet fuel rather than judging the quality of food on taste. When you look at a plate of food you're about to eat, think of this food in numbers and how will your body benefit from the meal. Think of a race car. Do you think the pit crew would fill up the tank with regular fuel instead of high-octane racing fuel? Absolutely not! So why wouldn't you eat "high-octane" food? That means lean protein, fiber from vegetables and fruit, and good fats all in the same meal. Try not to think of food and eating as just enjoyment. Instead, look at food as means to having a fantastic body and wonderful health.

Trust me, you can make that mental transition pretty easily. Once I did, everything else just fell into place. All of a sudden, looking good became much easier. What a relief that was! Getting in shape for the college wrestling season was a must for me. From October until April were never the easiest months. These months were tough, because the wrestling practices were grueling and I was constantly cutting weight in order to compete at the 190-pound division. The good news about those winter months is that I was forced into being in shape. At that point I began understanding that as a result of being on a college wrestling team, I was in shape for wrestling, not to look good. But as a result of being in wrestling shape, my body looked good, tight and lean. Because I really enjoyed wrestling and it got me into shape, why would I use a treadmill if I didn't enjoy it? Only to get into shape? All of a sudden my attitude toward fitness changed. I began to change my cardio workouts. Instead of treadmill work, I chose to do something that I liked, like playing my favorite sports. While in college my year was divided into two parts, wrestling season and summer. All winter long, even though wrestling practice and cutting weight were demanding, I still enjoyed it. The sacrifices, the commitment—this makes all the difference between being a champ or a chump. As soon as wrestling season ended, I would not workout or diet for one full week. After that week, I would be back to the grind of lifting weights and doing cardio. From mid-April until late September would be months of discipline for me to stay between 5 and 7 percent body fat with my weight at about 200 to 210 lbs. The winter mission was winning in wrestling and the summer mission was looking good for the beach.

Believe it or not, the summer months were much harder for me to maintain my shape than the winter. Why? Because I enjoyed wrestling and disliked treadmills, which was my summer cardio. Now I realized that in order to be in shape for the summer and not be grumpy half the time, I would need to incorporate fun cardio instead of treadmills. What did I do? I began playing soccer, tennis, wrestling and other sports I enjoyed. Not only were sports more fun for me, but I was gaining agility, both mental and physical. Most importantly, I was having a lot more fun. Looking good in the summer now became a breeze with that simple change.

The other part of having a nice body come with proper eating. Suddenly I felt an urgency to find more fun ways to diet instead of eating the same old diet food. I figured that if I can make that positive adjustment with my cardio, why can't this be done with my diet and weight lifting routine? That would make the process of getting into shape that much easier—and when it comes to getting into shape, any help possible is a huge advantage. Resistance training such as lifting weights or calisthenics would be next on my agenda to figure out which training methods would be the most enjoyable for me. I had been lifting weights on and off in the basement of my family's house since I was 14. On my 19th birthday I first walked into a weightlifting gym and paid for a year-long membership. From my 19th birthday I became 100 percent dedicated and showed it by working out five days per week.

For years, I trained in the same format, the one that everyone said is the best for gaining lean muscle mass. Notice that the word everyone is highlighted, because I now fell into the same category as most people do when they begin the process of getting into shape. I was doing what other people said was the best workout, even though there may have been another equally effective routine that would have been either better suited and or more enjoyable for me. Nevertheless, I continued to work out in the same manner even though the workouts were not that enjoyable. I continued because I definitely saw results. It wasn't until years later that I finally decided to start trying all different types of exercise routines. I wanted to test if they could actually be effective while I had more fun doing them. I tried calisthenics, barbells, dumbbells, doing 10 or 20 sets per body part, and training each body part once, twice or three times per week. Basically, I tried every possible combination that was available in my attempt to find a good resistance workout, one that I liked and could stick to without quitting.

The pattern of my past was I would start doing a workout routine that was recommended to me by another person who achieved positive results with that same workout. I would then train for several months, achieve nice results, then become completely bored with the exercise routine and end up stopping. This pattern plagued me for several years. Every time the workouts changed I hoped to find that one that I would like and not quit. Though trial and error, I eventually found resistance routines that I liked enough to want to continue without quitting. In my case, the routines that worked best for me, while at the same time being the easiest to continue without stopping, were all about variety. That meant changing my routines monthly, weekly or even daily. Frequently changing workouts was tailor-made for my lifestyle and personality. For a person like myself, who becomes bored rather quickly, nothing could be better than changing routines often. Now and for the last several years, my training has been pleasantly consistent, all thanks to finding the right workouts for me. Aside from changing the routines, I also found a new way to look at my workouts. Now I began using exercise to relieve stress, to put me into a better mood and to help me sleep better at night. These results are felt immediately! No longer was I working out only to look better physically. Now I was working out to make me feel better psychologically. It has been working great! Better than ever! Working out is so much better when you combine the physical with the psychological.

I still had one last obstacle to conquer—food. Eating right is so important, but at the same time the diet can be very bland and frustrating. Why not find a fun way to eat? Why not choose the healthy foods that you enjoy the most? Why not eat an apple instead of a pear if you like pears better? Why eat swordfish if you like red snapper better? Why not eat broccoli if you like it better than cauliflower? Why should you snack on almonds when you would rather have walnuts? Understand my concept? You can still choose which healthy foods to eat, because there are so many of them. This is exactly how I continue to eat healthy and stay in shape. Trust me, this is the secret to getting and keeping that nice body.. Keep it as fun as possible! Remember, time flies when you're having fun!

Chapter 20: In Shape Everywhere

Why not be fit everywhere and anywhere? It's really not that diffi-cult—I've been doing it for years. Wherever I may be, I always make sure to eat right and exercise even without the comfort of my home or gym. Public parks, hotel rooms, parking lots, fast-food, or high-end restaurants, there is a proper meal and workout available in all of these places. Regardless of the restaurant I can still eat healthy and regardless of my location I can still exercise properly. This is part of a larger picture. Quality of life begins with good health and confidence. We all agree that nobody wants to get old or be put of shape, right? Fortunately, I know how to counteract both with sim-ple changes in your life.

This book is the first in my series of easy-reading books. Each book is short, simple, to the point and specific about adapting your diet and workout to your desires. I wrote this book because I am 100 percent sure of my methods of getting into shape and maintaining your health, even if you are tied up in a hectic lifestyle. Please don't allow your health and body to suffer because of being away from home or the gym. Even though you are away from home, I can still help you attain the best shape of your life. The ultimate wealth is health, never forget this! Now let me guide you every step of the way toward developing the best body ever!

Chapter 21: The Best Investment Is Your Body

Whenever we think of the word "invest," we think of money and our future. Well, both are extremely important but so is a third investment—our health. This is the most important investment of all, because without health nothing else is possible. Investing in your health is a long-term commitment. You will not reap the benefits right away, but small changes in your everyday life will be noticed quickly. The changes may be small, but collectively they add up to improved quality of life. As we know, the ultimate happiness begins with the quality of life. That doesn't mean earning a huge salary, owning a beautiful house and car but hating going to work every day and being embarrassed by your body. Many people live in this predicament of being overworked in a run-down body.

I can change that, but only if you are willing to make the changes needed. By applying nutritional methods you will feel a sudden surge of energy and well-being. Yes! Nutrition is that important! Unfortunately, most people do not follow a healthy meal plan. They don't see diet as an important factor toward their happiness/quality of life. They couldn't be more misinformed! Eating properly is just as important as a good nights' sleep, and possibly more! It seems to me that quality of life is known understood by western Europeans. These people surely know how to live. My family's heritage is from Spain and I have been extremely fortunate to have spent many summers there. I learned so much by merely seeing how my cousins, uncles and friends lived. To them, a day was not complete without eating a well-balanced and fresh meal with the family, then taking a nap right after. To the typical western European work and money are not as important as quality food and rest. They must have a point because western Europeans have among the longest life spans in the world! And with a much lower obesity rate than the U.S! Why? Well ,for starters their diet consists of a lot of fish, red wine and salads. All important and nutritious food. Even more so, the western European culture is different—more of a quality, not quantity, mentality. These people take immense pride in what and how they eat. Isn't it a coincidence that western Europe as a whole is known for quality, including German cars, Italian fashion, and architecture. Most western European families prepare their own meals and rarely order fast food or take-out. That's how I want my clients to live, with home-cooked, balanced meals, like the Europeans. Custom-made Italian clothing with French cologne and driving a Porsche would be a nice touch as well!

In the next chapter I am going to teach you step 1, how to shop for food. We first need to build the foundation of a long-term relationship between ourselves and proper eating. Once you give me the chance to introduce you to a whole new world of healthy cooking and eating, you will never look back but only forward to health, happiness, positive energy and longevity! The rewards are priceless.

Chapter 22: Your Kitchen, Your Headquarters

Cooking healthy at home is only possible if the right ingredients are readily available in your refrigerator and pantry. This is extremely important. Avoid having triggers in your home, by which I mean any type of food or beverage that is not healthy. We're all human, so at any given time we can give in to temptation and cheat on our diets. Don't get me wrong! An occasional cheat meal is fine, but let's keep it occasional rather than frequent. If you have only the right foods in your home, it's much easier to stick to the diet.

Your pantry and refrigerator are at the heart of our quest to have the best body and health possible. Think of a race car. Doesn't a race car use premium fuel? OK, now you are the race car! In order to perform optimally, you need the best fuel possible, right? Well that fuel means eating fish, salads, whole-grain foods, and drinking plenty of water.

Food shopping is the first step toward having the best body and health imaginable. You can find all the foods you need in any chain supermarket. There's no need to shop at expensive health-food or specialty stores.

Food shopping for you will now change somewhat. The emphasis now more toward reading the product label to see the nutritional value instead of basing your choice on flavor, price, the attractiveness of the packaging, and so on. You can do this food shopping anywhere, even in a gas station convenience store.

Remember what I said about the western European culture of quality? Now we are going to start thinking about food along their terms, quality over quantity! To create the best body and health possible ,your kitchen will be starting point. Weekly trips to the supermarket will be common. Even though your supermarket bill may increase your food expenses everywhere else will decrease. Overall you will be spending less and you will look better and be healthier for less money! Great news!

Chapter 23: Let's Go Food Shopping

Having a kitchen stocked with nutritious food is extremely important. Supermarkets are the place to go for buying all of proper foods that will help you create the body you want and the health you need. Chain supermarkets are fine because plenty of fresh vegetables, fruits, fish, lean meats are always available. Weekly shopping for all of your food will provide you with all the fresh food you will need throughout the week.

Let's start with a typical walk down the aisles of your local supermarket.

Best Performance Foods

Advanced Level

Beverages:
Water, coffee, tea

Protein:
Skinless, boneless chicken breast
Skinless, boneless turkey breast
London broil
Eye round
Liquid egg whites
Omega-3 eggs
Wild-caught salmon (not farm-raised)
Canned tuna, salmon, sardines, mackerel

Whey isolate powder
Soy powder

Carbohydrates:
Sweet potatoes
Brown rice
Whole-grain pasta
Oat bran
Old-fashioned plain oats
Unprocessed wheat bran

Fiber:
Vegetables
Fruits

Fats:
Nuts
Olive oil
Canola oil
Avocados

I listed the best possible foods you could buy that would give your body its best look and health. However, some of these foods are not everyone's favorite, so I will also list more foods you can buy that may be a little more common for everyday eating. This list of intermediate level foods is more taste friendly and common for family dinners or inviting guests over to eat. With these foods, you can still enjoy eating with only minor changes to your cooking. When I invite friends or family over for dinner, I am not about to serve steamed chicken. Broiled chicken breast with olive oil and lemon would be more suitable for everyone.

Intermediate Level

Protein:
Lean chicken breast
Lean turkey breast
Lean pork cuts
Sirloin
Skirt steak
All fish and seafood are acceptable.

Carbohydrates:
Red potatoes
Wild rice
Quick oatmeal
Quinoa
Whole-wheat pasta
Nonfat Greek yogurt
Bran cereal

Fibers:
Frozen vegetables
Frozen fruits

Fats:
All-natural peanut butter (unsalted)
All-natural almond butter (unsalted)

The intermediate diet food shopping list is in addition to the advanced list. Shop as if you are an advanced dieter. You want to eventually ease from the intermediate to the advanced level in such a subtle way that you won't even notice! That's the secret of success with this—ease your way into the advanced level so you won't notice any drastic changes. The better you eat, the better you will feel, I will

promise this!
Beginner Level

Protein:
Chicken
Turkey breast,
Lean cuts of pork
 90 percent lean ground beef
All fish and seafood

Carbohydrates :
White Potatoes
Long-grain rice
Sugar-free flavored instant oatmeal

Fats:
Peanut butter

Fibers:
Canned vegetables (unsalted)
Canned fruits (unsweetened)

As a beginner you should also buy the intermediate and advanced foods as well so you can occasionally sneak them into your beginner's meals.

I've just given you a pretty detailed list of the foods that you should be buying, whether you are a beginner, intermediate and advanced. Of course, eating out occasionally is to be expected. Check back to section II of this book for healthier alternatives on the menu.

My true goal is to see you make subtle improvements, nothing drastic. I have learned that slow, subtle improvements have a higher long-term success ratio than attempting drastic changes. Sudden dietary changes in an attempt to look great for an event like a wedding that will be happening soon don't work and damage your health. Remember, creating a great body is a marathon, not a sprint. As much as I would love to tell you that in no time at all you will look great, I would be lying if I did. This is a slow process, but fortunately you will still notice improvements on practically a daily basis! You will have so much fun seeing yourself slowly but surely change for the better! Of course, I enjoy seeing my own progress but I am so excited as well seeing the progress of others using my body transforming methods. Whenever my clients say "Thanks, Chris, for helping me improve my body," I am ecstatic! My clients' improvements are so rewarding for me, I am so happy whenever I see this!

Chapter 24: Kitchen Tools and Appliances

In chapter 23 I just explained which foods to buy when food shopping. Of course, the foods are very important, but so are the tools, utensils and appliances that will be used for food preparation and cooking. Buying these items may sound like a serious commitment, but not really. They're not that expensive, they last a long time and they make a big difference in being able to prepare the right foods easily. I am able to prepare nutritious gourmet meals quickly and efficiently, with minimal mess and clean-up time! Whenever I invite people over to eat, they are always amazed, for several reasons. For starters, they are very impressed with how great the food tastes without even knowing that they are eating a low-calorie, healthy meal! Also, they are amazed with how quickly it was all prepared. They are finishing up with dessert and tea without even realizing that I already quickly cleaned up all the dishes, pots, etc. Then they finally realize that it was a healthy, low-calorie, dietetic meal. How? Because three hours later, they felt light, energetic and even hungry again! Those are the telltale signs of healthy eating: feeling light and energetic after eating with no sluggish feeling and downtime after and a few hours later feeling hungry again! That means your body already burned through that meal and your metabolism is increasing as a result. An increased metabolism is what we all want, because it keeps you revved and alert while your body burns more calories throughout the day. An increased metabolism helps you burn more fat and allows you to eat more calories! That right there is the magic bullet!

Kitchen Tools and Appliances
Food scale
Measuring cup
Strainer
Electric or manual steamer
Sealable quart- and gallon-sized plastic food storage bags
Plastic food storage containers in various sizes

The food scale and measuring cup are absolutely necessary for portion control. You would be surprised how crucial it is to measure your portions in order to create that beautiful physique. One extra ounce more or less can be the difference between making or breaking your entire physique! Seems crazy, doesn't it? But based on own experience of being a competitive champion bodybuilder, Golden Gloves boxer and NCAA two-time All-American college wrestler, I know this is 100 percent true. In these sports, optimally adjusting and measuring body weight and body fat is the difference between winning and losing. You also need food storage containers. They're important because they improve cooking efficiency. Whenever I cook, I always prepare several meals at once. Cooking one or three of the same meal takes the same amount of time. Now that you will be eating every two to four hours, you don't want to cook five times a day. Instead, cook once or twice for ten to fifteen minutes and store the food in Ziploc storage bags or plastic container. That way, you have healthy prepared meals accessible all day long. This increases time and energy efficiency. Less time, less electricity, less gas used! Sounds like a winning proposition!

Chapter 25: Quick Healthy Recipes

Now let's put everything together: healthy food, well-stocked kitchen and all the tools and appliances needed to create the meals necessary to improve your body, energy and health. I apologize for taking so long to finally get to this chapter of recipes and meals. The previous chapters provided the proper foundation toward success in creating the body you want with optimum health. Yes, it would be so much easier for me to simply write out a bunch of simple recipes and then say "good luck" and send you on your way. But I thrive when my clients results and I see results. It's extremely gratifying! That's the same feeling I get when coaching wrestling. As a volunteer wrestling coach, when I see my athletes succeed and know that my own knowledge played even a minor role in their success, it's an unbelievably gratifying sensation. The feeling of giving back is extremely satisfying. Never will I forget the people who made a positive impact in my life. I'm extremely grateful to them. The cycle of giving and receiving must continue on a daily basis—plus it makes you feel great!

Once again I will give examples of body-improving recipes and meals for the beginner, intermediate and advanced. You will be able to see video recordings of how the meals are prepared as well to help further assist you in achieving your goals of fitness and health.

Believe it or not, preparing top-quality nutritious meals is really simple and has nothing but positive benefits. If there are meal combinations that you would like but don't see them listed here, I would be more than happy to upgrade the list. I want to better accommodate you with a wider variety of meals to help facilitate the process of achieving that body you want!

Beginner: Complete Day of Power-Packed Meals

Breakfast (7 A.M.)

Option 1:
1/2 cup egg whites, 1 whole omega 3 egg
1 packet sugar-free flavored instant oatmeal

For the eggs, spray cooking oil (Pam) onto frying pan (2- to 3-second spray is sufficient). Heat pan, then pour egg whites and crack entire omega 3 egg into frying pan. Cook for a few minutes, then flip over for another minute or so until cooked through.

For the oatmeal, pour contents of packet into a bowl and add hot water or place in microwave oven for 2 minutes or so (follow packet directions if in doubt).

Option 2:
1 scoop whey protein isolate
1 apple
Ice cubes
Cinnamon

Pour whey protein isolate, apple, ice cubes and cinnamon to taste into a blender. Blend on high until ice is completely broken up.

Mid-morning snack (10 A.M.)

Option 1:
1 cup nonfat plain Greek yogurt

Option 2:
1 fruit

Lunch (1 P.M.)

Option 1:
Low-sodium turkey breast sandwich on whole-grain bread with mustard, lettuce and tomato

Option 2:
1 can light tuna in water
Mixed green salad with oil and vinegar dressing

Mid-afternoon snack (4 P.M.)

Option1:
1 plain fruit cocktail

Option 2:
2 ounces (1 packet) unsalted nuts

Dinner (7 P.M.)

Option 1:
6 ounces London broil
Steamed vegetables

Option 2:
6 ounces broiled fish
Steamed vegetables

Bedtime snack (around 10 p.m. only if you are hungry)

Option 1:
1 cup low-fat plain cottage cheese

Option 2:
2 tablespoons peanut butter

There you have it, a full day of properly balanced meals for the beginner who wants to change his body and health for the better. The meals are simple to follow and prepare. As you grow into this meal plan, you will start to see positive changes in your appearance and feeling of well-being. You will want to make a few minor adjustments over time. You might change the times you eat or how many meals and snacks you eat throughout the day. You are beginning a journey toward having a better body and health!

Intermediate: Complete Day of Power-Packed Meals

Breakfast (7 A.M.)

Option 1:
2/3 cup liquid egg whites, 1 whole omega 3 egg
½ cup plain old-fashioned oatmeal
1 fruit

Option 2:
2/3 cup quinoa
1 scoop whey protein isolate

To prepare quinoa, rinse it first in cold water. Place in large bowl and add 2 cups water. Microwave for 3 minutes. Stir in whey isolate powder. Note: Pronounced KEEN-wa, quinoa is a high-protein, high-fiber grain from the Andes. It makes a good substitute for rice, pasta, and potatoes.

Mid-morning snack (10 A.M.)

Option 1:
2 tablespoons almond butter

Option2:
1 fruit

Lunch (1P.M.)

Option1:
1 can or pouch salmon in water, mixed with lettuce, tomato, cucumber, vinegar and oil

Option 2:
6 ounces 90% lean broiled beef patty on high fiber bun with lettuce and tomato

Mid-afternoon snack or pre-workout meal (4 P.M.)

Option 1:
1 fruit with 1 tablespoon peanut butter

Option 2:
1 scoop whey protein isolate with 1 banana

Dinner or post-workout meal (7 p.m.)

Option 1:
6 ounces grilled fish
Sautéed vegetables
1 cup sliced fresh fruit

Preparation: Grill fish in skillet with garlic, tomatoes and string beans.

Option 2:
6 ounces fresh turkey breast grilled with onions
Whole-wheat pita bread
Green salad
1 cup fresh strawberries

Bedtime snack (around 10 P.M. only if you are hungry)

Option 1:
5 hard-boiled egg whites, 1 hard-boiled egg yolk

Option 2:
1 can octopus in water

The intermediate meal plan involves a bit more cooking and is more involved Please don't be intimidated! It's easy to follow—and I can change it in so many ways to make it even easier for you. The results you will see in your body will speak for themselves! Totally! A great body is priceless! And in such high demand! We all want to be lean, healthy and proud each time we look in the mirror!

Advanced: Complete Day of Power-Packed Meals

Early-morning cardio for 30 minutes

Breakfast (7 A.M.)
¾ cup liquid egg whites, 1 whole omega 3 egg
1 high-fiber pancake

Pancake preparation: Mix 1 cup pancake batter with water until smooth. Spray frying pan with oil. Add batter when pan is hot. When bubbles form on top of pancake, flip over and cook other side until lightly browned.

Option 2:
1½ scoops whey protein isolate blended with ice
½ cup old-fashioned oats
1 small fruit
7 almonds

Mid-morning snack (10 A.M.)

Option 1:
1 apple
8 walnuts

Option 2:
2 tablespoons all-natural peanut butter

Lunch (1 P.M.)

Option 1:
1 high-fiber tortilla wrap with 1 can light tuna in water; season with mustard

Option 2:
1 hard-boiled egg and 1/3-pound sliced turkey on 2 slices high-fiber whole-grain bread; season with vinegar

Mid-afternoon snack or pre-workout meal (4 P.M.)

Option 1:
1 tablespoon all-natural almond butter

1 fruit

Option 2:
1 can sardines in water mixed with 1 cup brown rice
Dinner or post-workout meal (7p.m.)

Option1:
6 ounces steamed salmon
1 cup whole-grain pasta
Steamed vegetables

Preparation: Place salmon and vegetables in steamer and cook together for about 20 minutes.

Option 2:
6 ounces broiled sirloin steak
Green salad with oil and vinegar dressing
Sugar-free Jell-O

Bedtime snack (around 10 p.m. only if you are hungry)

Option 1:
1 can or pouch salmon in water combined with chopped cucumber and onions, seasoned with vinegar

Option 2:
¾ cup egg whites sprinkled with non-fat cheese

The advanced meal plan is just another simple step up. This level will render dramatic improvements not only in the look of your body but your mental and physical health as well. Believe it or not, your brain's cognitive functions also improves. Your mind will be sharper, you'll feel more alert and have a clearer memory!

I've listed just a few examples of different meals in this chapter. As I have said before, many, many more options exist. The food choices are endless! This is a proven method that really works by improving your body and mind!

The first step is always the hardest, but once it's taken you will experience a revelation! You will witness improvements across the board, from your appearance to your attitude. Everything will be better!

Chapter 26: Implementing the Strategy

The start is always the most difficult challenge whenever we implement a new game plan. Those of you who have dieted and exercised before know that we are forever seeking that magic bullet of a workout and diet that's effortless but renders dramatic results. Well, I am still searching for that Easy Way Out, but so far I haven't found it. After all my years of competitive sports, nutrition and training I have come to the conclusion that the magic bullet is commitment.

The good news is that with every passing year I find better ways to make looking good easier and easier. I have come to a point where following my methods of training and dieting is much easier than just living an average life. When you're not dieting or training you lose your zest, the spark in life that drives us to be active and reach our goals. Whenever I slack off on training and dieting, I end up slacking off on life in general. I end up missing opportunities because I don't feel like going for that bike ride, or that friend's BBQ, or playing with kids, or playing my musical instruments. Understand what I mean? When I am in shape—eating and training properly— my mind and body are at 110 percent. I'm loaded with firepower! That makes me want to go bike riding, clean the garage, go to that social event, invite friends over to play soccer, mow my neighbor's lawn or do anything else that's productive and physical. Once you're in shape, your mind opens to the next level, making productivity and happiness go hand in hand.

Training increases opportunity and lessens fear of rejection. It lets you go for that hidden dream, the one you're embarrassed to tell people about. Following my methods is not just about looking better—that's just the tip of the iceberg! My methods are about being better! So please, understand that life is short, and youth is even shorter! Why not stay young for as long as we can, for as long as we are willing to commit? Follow my system of life improvement and youth will be a part of your life, even if your age says otherwise! Youth is positive energy and strength. Why not have this always? It can be done! Believe and you shall achieve!

www.ingramcontent.com/pod-product-compliance
Lightning Source LLC
Chambersburg PA
CBHW050533280326
41933CB00011B/1565